Omad

Easy & Quick Leads Recipes to Attain Weight Loss

(An Essential Guide to One Meal a Day Intermittent Fasting With Simple)

Leslie Dimarco

Published By **Oliver Leish**

Leslie Dimarco

Omad: Easy & Quick Leads Recipes to Attain Weight Loss (An Essential Guide to One Meal a Day Intermittent Fasting With Simple)

ISBN   978-1-998901-42-5

No part of this guidebook shall be reproduced in any form without permission in writing from the publisher except in the case of brief quotations embodied in critical articles or reviews.

Legal & Disclaimer

The information contained in this ebook is not designed to replace or take the place of any form of medicine or professional medical advice. The information in this ebook has been provided for educational & entertainment purposes only.

The information contained in this book has been compiled from sources deemed reliable, and it is accurate to the best of the Author's knowledge; however, the Author cannot guarantee its accuracy and validity and cannot be held liable for any errors or omissions. Changes are periodically made to this book. You must consult your doctor or get professional medical advice before using

Table Of Contents

Chapter 1: Lose 4-10 Pounds Immediately (Phase 1)

Want a brief weight loss plan? Here it's far. Lose four-10 kilos proper now.

1. One of the fastest techniques to shed pounds is through fasting. I am no longer telling you to not consume something for each week, but if you may, skip dinner or breakfast. If you may do it for every week or , you will lose four-10 kilos in your first month. It befell so rapid and I out of place plenty weight! However, I had not a few issue to fear because of the fact I changed into eating sufficient meals and I felt locate it impossible to resist too. I even have grow to be hungry, however I have to experience that my belly modified into getting smaller and flatter. My waistline come to be getting smaller, my glide changed into better with ldl cholesterol degree barely taking place, and my liver

(GOP and GTP) degrees progressed fast too.

2. Beginner's proper fortune, in case you have a look at Paulo Coelho's novel, "The Alchemist" you simply understand what I suggest. It is a God given gift for starters taking over a private legend or a life prolonged adventure to find out treasure. In our case, it is probably fulfillment in weight-reduction plan. It is your first jackpot in a lottery or your first win in a chance. I dare say you need to revel in it whilst it lasts.

3. Why? Because it quickly scares you. True, triumphing with masses of opportunities worried scares humans in a while. Trust me; food plan has greater to do along with your thoughts than some thing else does. Unless you're huge, fats, or overweight because of clinical reasons, then it's far mainly because of your intellectual and social topics. If you win as

soon as and keep to win without an lousy lot attempt, you may rapid count on that it's far dull. Diet is in no manner like that. We understand how tough it's far. Especially while you age, it only receives more difficult to shed pounds. It is much like life, it tremendous receives tougher to combat. You may probably as nicely enjoy it on the same time as you're nice.

four. Actually, the number one time I misplaced weight via fasting, passed off once I became in high university. It have grow to be my first weight loss program and I had to fast for one week. I did not consume for 3 days and I out of area weight so fast that it scared me. If you're extra younger, the impact of fasting is greater due to the fact your metabolism is better. However, after 3 days I have been given scared. I had already out of place 10 kilos through then, and I lost my urge for meals too. For the primary days, I did now not eat a few aspect. Only at the 0.33 day did I drink a few water. I idea I might also additionally die, so I slowly commenced out ingesting another time with porridge. My stomach harm a piece, however I quickly recovered. My weight shot up once more as fast as I commenced out eating over again.

5. So, what's my thing? Don't be afraid of the bodily modifications. If you had a weight loss program earlier than, you gained't be scared. If this is your first time, you might be scared after dropping masses weight indoors days, weeks, or possibly months. The impact is brilliant inside the beginning. Enjoy it even because it lasts. Think simply, specially whilst your body conditions decorate. Your frame will cherish it, and so will you. It is a blessing and it's miles awesome!

6. If this is your first time happening a weight loss plan, it is able to be tough on

the way to bypass food or to eat small quantities. I despite the fact that find it especially hard to devour smaller amounts in step with meal at the same time as there may be a loads of food to devour. My stomach grumbles as a signal that I want extra meals. However, you have to learn how to recognize even as your frame starts to shed pounds. Every morning you awaken feeling your belly getting flatter and hungry that is an illustration you're dropping weight. Every morning you wake up feeling lousy and seem to have a glide trouble this is an alarm, you're gaining weight.

7. One very important key to achievement in a eating regimen is sustainability. Is your weight loss plan sustainable and for how lengthy? I couldn't deal with my fashionable fasting in excessive university for extra than three days. I knew I ought to in truth lose some weight, but I gave up

due to the fact I knew I couldn't rapid for all time.

8. Another important key to achievement in a weight loss plan is your adaptability. What may also you do even as you wake up at 1 or 3am inside the morning because of the reality you're hungry? This will sincerely take area to most people while we begin skipping dinner. How may additionally need to you adjust some time table to be more effective on the identical time as you skip meals? What would possibly you do for the loose hours you get?

nine. The moment people recognize some element terrible is going to take vicinity, they have a tendency to give up. Well, that's terrible. My trick isn't always to apply any trick. Just be honest to yourself. Work on a way that honestly works. Believe in it and stay your life the manner you designed it. It truely works!

10. To sum up, bypass your breakfast or dinner. Skipping dinner (save you consuming in advance than six pm) works great. It is a quick, healthful manner of dropping weight. Skipping breakfast doesn't art work so nicely, however works as a exquisite accelerator at the same time as you do it with skipping dinner. Drink severa water to replenish your starvation. Do this for one month. I weighed 202 pounds after I began out. Then, I out of place 15pounds in a unmarried month (four weeks)! Good genuine fortune!

Email me approximately your fulfillment story after your first month weight reduction. What is your name? Where are you from? How many kilos (or kg) did you lose on your first month? Are you glad? What's your subsequent intention? I may be reached at thelifesuccess1@gmail.Com.

Chapter 2: Fight Your Hunger (Phase 2)

Here is my thriller to healthy eating plan achievement. You are about to have interaction in a cutting-edge manner of life.

1. Let me let you know what I do. I am a researcher/instructor and characteristic a Ph.D. However not a medical diploma. Therefore, I am a mean individual near diet. I am in my early forties. My accomplice is a nutritionist (with a Ph.D.) but she and I stay on unique diets. She eats three very small meals a day with snacks and espresso. I on opposite consume one meal an afternoon.

2. This form of difference is without a doubt very commonplace among practitioners. Dr. Nagumo Yoshinori's partner or his distinct own family contributors don't exercise what he does and the own family actually works great. I too, have youngsters and I don't inform

them to head on my diet as they're too younger. I assume one should be at least two many years vintage or older to exercise weight loss plan. This new software program can be your buddy all of the time.

three. I take multi-nutrients and eating regimen C (1000mg) each day. I do no longer take any remedy. I weigh myself greater than three instances an afternoon (times within the morning and as quickly as at night time) with a health club outstanding weight scale ($three hundred or greater) and maintain facts of my body fat and muscle mass.

four. In the morning, I drink one or warmth cups of thick almond milk, soymilk or milk. I now and again add numerous freshly ground toasted plants (sesame seeds, black beans, soybeans, perilla seeds, sticky rice, rice, brown rice, oats or another exceptional grain mixes), but this is not critical. I eat one or two bars of chocolate (34g every). It may be dark chocolate or milk chocolate, however I try and stay with one specific emblem this is effectively available. That way I can effects depend the strength and hold my food plan everywhere I tour.

five. In terms of the energy for my breakfast, bars of chocolate and two cups of heat milk is identical to as a minimum one mild meal on the identical time as we depend the strength. However, it is better than bacons, sausages, ham and eggs or a whole meal (breakfast buffet at a inn) as it does not make you experience tired. Liquid diet regime works because of the reality beverages do not drain your energy not like strong factors. This way, you can use the unused electricity in digesting immoderate power that in the long run receives stored for your body as fat.

6. Throughout the day, to combat my starvation, I drink loads of numerous warmth non-caffeinated crop-based totally definitely tea, which consist of barley, corn, and others, normally as tons as half a gallon (1-2 liters). Warm beverages maintain your body temperature warmth, assisting you to burn extra calories. Crop primarily based definitely tea preserve you healthy and keeps your belly complete more than water. You can boil it with less water and may drink it thick, however it although has little or no calories. I may moreover drink black tea, green tea once in a while, but I do not drink coffee in any respect.

7. I eat lunch at noon and may consume some aspect any quantity I need. In the beyond, I used to pile up meals and eat like loopy. My lunch varies in keeping with what my frame desires. I can eat seafood, pork or vegetables. Usually, I consume

many particular types of meals. I strive no longer to fill my full meal with one severe trouble or . I try to keep away from eating donuts, goodies, sweets, fatty meals, or greasy food to extremes. I can try this however consciously.

8. After lunch, I take a 30 min. To one-hour nap. I usually do no longer devour dinner but try to accommodate friends and myself for brilliant sports. If this is the case, I bypass lunch and eat dinner as an opportunity. These days are fairly difficult so I drink juice or tea to maintain myself less hungry. This commonly takes region as quickly as per week or as speedy as a month. You want in case you want to change your mealtime from time to time to make your food regimen sustainable.

9. Usually I go to mattress early spherical 10 or 11pm on an empty stomach. My modern-day bedtime is middle of the night. I crash on an empty belly. When I

am hungry and can not get to sleep because of that, I drink barley tea or drink water and I sleep like a toddler. I wake up in the morning feeling honestly rejuvenated. I eat pleasant one complete meal a day.

10. Most articles that I even have have a look at on durability all seem to say that folks that stay close to a hundred or greater every consume one meal an afternoon, meals a day or 3 moderate meals a day. None of them eats to extremes. They furthermore preserve their meal times efficiently. These people are also proper at maintaining a healthy healthy eating plan for a long term and so should we.

eleven. You can't use too many versions on what you could consume. For example, you cannot truely add or subtract what you consume for at the least first or three months. If you eat many one of a kind varieties of food, you most effective confuse your frame. This can be very critical. If you exchange what you eat, you are strain. Therefore, you want to move regular till your frame gets used to it. Trust me it takes time weeks or months to tame your body to observe your lead. Do no longer permit it panic through often converting your food plan. Go constant at the begin and slowly experiment and alternate what you eat.

12. To sum it up, that permits you to make it a lifestyles lengthy food plan, you want to perform a little element that is sustainable. I do liquid weight loss plan within the morning and devour one full meal a day. I drink one to 2 cups of warm soymilk or milk with powdered plants, and consume a chocolate bar or . When I simply have dinner dates, I drink juices or tea within the afternoon and eat dinner. I visit mattress early round 10pm. First,

popularity on happening a consistent diet plan.

Chapter 3: Cheating Is Okay

Cheating is okay as long as you understand what it does. Cheat simplest when you have to. And whilst you cheat, use it on your benefit.

Obviously, you do not need to cheat, if you are this kind of robust willed character. I do not have a strong will. I am a median man or woman with regards to food. Actually, I love food and that is why I could not attain success in my weight loss program for a long term. However, I even have located numerous strategies to use dishonest to my benefit.

1. When do I cheat? I used to cheat hundreds inside the first three months. Now, I without a doubt do not cheat the least bit, because of the reality I do not have any motive to. Of path, after I do

cheat, I recall the strength. In the morning, as soon as I am hungry, I drink cups of warm milk in place of 1. If I can not wait till lunch, I devour chocolate bars (of the identical logo) in desire to at least one. I drink crop-based tea extra often.

2. I actually have a massive Japanese tea thermos (1gallon/2.2 liters) in my office and freshly brew crop based tea at the least as quickly as a day. I continuously surround myself with diverse varieties of tea to keep myself a whole lot a lot less hungry. Sometimes, once I am on a lunch date and do not devour enough, I want to consume greater after the dinner to fill my empty belly. If you do now not fill up your stomach, snacking for the duration of the day is recommended.

three. However, there may be one real DONT. That is snacking at night time. This is some component I now not frequently ever did. Eating late or consuming inside the nighttime is a few issue you should absolutely keep away from. Whether you noticed this on TV or what, it's far very awful and it ruins your diet plan. This can also furthermore stress you to begin all all over again. This is likewise some issue that I genuinely have never finished in my complete exercising. The key to achievement isn't always to eat after 6pm.

four. When I cheated, I gave myself a restriction. That became multiple times every week, in no way three instances. Sometimes over the weekend whilst families gather, I commonly attempt to have family gatherings for lunch instead of dinner, because of the reality then, I couldn't should starve until dinnertime. Nowadays, I do now not like eating dinner, however own family conditions pressure you to spend time with them, proper? The time is so treasured that you need to charge the possibility and in fact revel in it.

5. So, on the same time as sudden circle of relatives gatherings took place, I ended up consuming dinner. Therefore, I might devour lunch and dinner. Sometimes once I were given up very hungry, I should consume for me to sleep. I did breakfast and lunch. I ate lots decrease back then. However, I in no way gorged myself 3 whole meals. Usually, one meal (each lunch or dinner) have grow to be full, and the opposite have become greater of a snack. I simply ate some component very mild to fill my stomach. I did that for 3 months.

6. After the fourth month, I may also need to in truth stick with my one meal food regimen. I knew and my frame knew what would possibly seem if I cheated. I would probably have a "very terrible" sleep in place of "superb" sleep. I need to in reality evaluate the two. Slowly, I actually have

emerge as remote from "very terrible" sleep. It have become high-quality.

7. Another benefit that I found from those cheatings emerge as at my scientific checkups. After numerous months, my stages have been now not enhancing in any respect. When I took the blood test at the medical institution, all my other tiers (liver, blood pressure, and the rest) were down, but my weight and my cholesterol levels had been no longer decreasing the least bit. Only then did I understand that I had to do something positive about it.

8. As you still sleep with an empty belly at night time time, you progressively lower your belly length and you may quality eat plenty an awful lot less as days go with the aid of. Therefore, in place of eating cups of heat milk, I have to devour most effective one. Then, in place of cheating, I have to in reality consume the chocolate

once I come to be noticeably hungry inside the afternoon.

nine. Now, the fine gain of you taking matters slowly is that your expectancies are restrained. Unlike the primary month on the same time as you enjoyed a excellent thrill in losing a variety of weight, the change is truly slower, but it takes location little by little. It is a top notch feeling and a stable one. Because, even as you continue to shed pounds at such an improved pace, you can begin to fear about your fitness, and you may start to eat again. You will regain your weight over again.

10. From your 2nd or zero.33 month, assume to lose handiest 4 kilos a month. That is only a pound in step with week. In addition, you can enjoy weight fluctuations. This takes place as you drink pretty some water. Water permits you together collectively along with your pass

and cleanses your tool. The much less you consume, the cleaner your tool gets. Do now not be disappointed.

eleven. To sum it up, dishonest is ok so long as you recognize what you are doing. Cheat nice to get by, and in no manner to overdo anything. Only snack while you're hungry for the duration of the day, and in no way past due at night time time. Fully experience your one entire meal within the path of the day. Eat only to fill the starvation. Try to get with the useful resource of your day until you nod off. Once you doze off, it's far any other win. This is how you win. You take small victories till you get accustomed to them. Later, you could add on to your preceding victories.

Chapter 4: Truly Understand Yoyo

Weigh yourself as a minimum three times an afternoon and apprehend what yoyo is all approximately.

There are three levels to this diet. Once you get used to as a minimum one meal a day workout (phase 3), you need to often gradual down on your dependancy of overeating. Overeating is in no way accurate. Eat lunch to your satisfaction and fill your stomach. Then, whilst you are hungry, snack within the past due afternoon (in case you do not need to, you do now not must). This is wiser and greater healthy. Eating or 3 small food a day is first rate so long as you don't overeat. Many individuals who live up to greater than 100 workout this.

1. Why is it essential to weigh at the least three instances an afternoon? To understand the load variations, the motives of weight losses or earnings, and

take benefit or the yo-yo. I usually begin my day early like around 5 or six inside the morning. That is everyday for a primitive guy like me.

2. The first detail I do is to weigh myself on the dimensions. I nearly flow into nude to get an accurate size. Then, I drink a cup of barley tea or a glass of water and get to paintings in my pc, watching for my frame's bathroom signal.

three. After doing my primary or in rest room, I weigh myself on the scale one more time. I get the difference. The distinction is massive! Usually, I lose 1 / four of a pound after number 1 or one or two kilos after quantity 2. Now, that is your actual weight with not anything on your stomach. Take a photograph of your weight as a record.

4. Even in spite of the reality that this is optionally to be had, I every now and then

weigh myself after lunch clearly to appearance how loads I received for lunch. Then, after returning home from paintings in the midnight, I weigh myself for the 1/3 time. This of course, I do once I go to the bathroom. Now, how a good buy do you weigh? You might also in all likelihood weigh extra. It is ok. This is a yo-yo and it is a cycle.

5. You consume and your weight will boom. If you consume greater than you eat, your weight decreases. Your body doesn't tell a lie. Make it honest. That manner, you can test collectively along with your meals and studies extra about the motives of weight loss and advantage. If you ate too much of a few component, felt superb, and didn't benefit weight, that's remarkable. However, in case you ate little or no and despite the fact that gained lots, that's now not unique. As you

have got got were given guessed, the oily, candy, or salty food makes you fat.

6. Also, spare it gradual to get recommendation from a health expert. When your frame is sincere, your health professionals' (nutritionist, medical clinical physician) advice works high-quality. As they see brilliant adjustments to your body, they will attempt that will help you extra. Be sincere to yourself and to your health experts.

7. To sum it up, you want to weigh yourself on the size at least 3 to four times a day. That manner you will be aware body weight fluctuations relying at the time of day, and earlier than and after meals. This manner, you may train your thoughts and body to speak absolutely.

Chapter 5: Train Your Body To Tell The Truth

Your body can take almost something even as you are young and healthy. What you have got is a buffer.

1. Of course, you could train your frame to lie. Our frame device is so clever that it lies and you won't even understand it. You pay hobby thin human beings brag about gorging immoderate calorie beverages or meals the opportunity every day and declare they did not gain any weight. They count on it's miles a heroic story, however I call it an risky story.

2. If you without a doubt recognize how an lousy lot your frame does to assist your device, your horrible consuming and slumbering conduct, you will be surprised at its resilience and enhancing capability. However, a number of those structures of yours in the end runs down over the years and you may quick be left with an vintage

house with leaking roof, damaged home windows, and a rickety door. This can also additionally sound sad, but it's far the final reality. We all stay to run our very structures down. Some do it faster at the same time as others do it slower.

three. I truly have a unhappy tale of a seventy 4 years vintage diabetic affected individual, who has been on a completely strict diet regime for the past thirty years thinking about his first diagnosis. Every time I dine with him, I expect he's an ascetic, however he although does not call himself a terrific ascetic. He says he however cheats once in a while. One day he shared his tale with me of the way and what he ate in his young adults and it went like this.

four. Everyday, he had 5 cans of soda, ate hamburgers, ice cream and desserts for cakes, meat, meat soup, and barbecues and alcohol at night time. However, he although awakened and went to paintings tomorrow. It have become hard for him, however he did it for 2 many years.

five. At first, he did not gain any weight, so he persevered the dependancy for five to ten years. His buffer began to wear down early. When you are younger and wholesome, you have got were given were given an splendid buffer location that would assist your crazy lifestyle. You don't appear to benefit any weight after a night time time of heavy booze, food, and partying.

6. If you do that sometimes, then your buffer recovers slowly. The restoration may be days, weeks or months. Remember that this "buffer" is a very summary time period and all people's specific frame situations are specific and particular. Just like how some human beings are born robust and whilst some are born prone.

7. If you are born wholesome, your organ simplest fails on the equal time as you abuse it. Once you deplete all your buffers, then, you come to be inclined. While the buffer is active, your body can inform a lie. Once you bypass that bodily buffer (or your restriction), you switch out to be persistent. You enjoy fatigue every morning, your frame aches, and you have were given issues in your stomach, coronary coronary heart, pores and pores and skin, liver, and circulate.

eight. On pinnacle of all this, you act advise to others. You have an effect on the lives of these near you negatively. You come to be dangerous and propose man or woman or a great-natured obese man or woman.

nine. Going decrease lower back to our story, this vintage guy's buffer changed into wiped out. The medical doctor knowledgeable him that his ldl cholesterol degree, GOP, and GTP had been off the charts. His pancreas modified into no longer functioning properly. It modified into damaged down for appropriate and will never be constant. Ever because of the fact then, he has been on a strict weight-reduction plan with remedy. When do you recognise the fee of lifestyles or happiness? Only even as you begin to lose it.

10. A new definition of health: You sense first rate normal you wake up, you haven't any troubles, you're free of pains, and persistent illnesses. Your clinical report says you are healthy and ordinary. You sleep like a infant at night time time, and you have were given a very thick buffer for life's struggles and barriers, which may furthermore get up at any time. Your life is with out primary worries of finance, device, relationships, and private existence. You are active, and you're

outstanding to yourself and to others. You are inclined to take risks and do no longer abuse your frame in any way. You revel in like you've got got the next day.

11. The smaller you're taking, the greater you get to revel in existence and the little matters. Lengthen the a laugh and leisure via taking smaller bites out of food and life. When I first started this healthy eating plan, I ate like loopy. I had a hard and fast aim, I awakened, and I filled my mouth with chocolate and soymilk. Then, I may also fear until lunch, quality to stuff myself with an in depth quantity of food. Now, I not do this. I fine consume pretty despite the fact that I great devour as soon as a day. It is flawlessly great for me. One meal an afternoon is enough to run you through the complete day and night time, now not to mention it assist you to relaxation.

12. During your first week, you may shed pounds hastily. However, do not panic.

During my first week, I out of place 10 pounds and I have emerge as scared. I idea some thing terrible changed into going to take place however most effective well things took place. My weight continuously reduced whilst my stamina (buffer) started to growth. I might also want to paintings longer hours and sleep plenty much less. I have to recognition higher. However, there has been one drawback. I felt like I did no longer have enough electricity.

13. The reality of the matter is that you get energy improve while you overeat. It gets you excessive and also you get a spike on your chart. However, hitting excessive manner you'll soon hit the deeper valley, which usually eventually finally ends up in a crash. Sugar crash, exhaustion, horrible motion, and liver failure are exceptional few of those symptoms and symptoms and signs that I can with out problems call. In

different phrases, hitting excessive is in no manner specific. It does now not assist.

14. Energy boosts and stimulants are not right. Just learn how to take subjects slowly and regularly, moderation is the form of existence. When you overeat, your liver and belly over characteristic, getting rid of most of the blood and strength from extraordinary organs, making you revel in lousier.

15. If you are continuously binging, consuming, and consuming, whilst does your body ever relaxation? You truly do no longer. You need to located your frame to relaxation through now not consuming. By decreasing the extensive sort of meals regular with day, you could moreover recognition greater on paintings and get more subjects completed. Yes, there may be a whole lot much less extemporaneous fun, however greater balance and strength

and buffers. The greater the buffer, the more wholesome you are.

16. To sum up, you want to devour pretty and take matters slowly. Overeating is never well. When it consists of consuming conduct, you located you are converting one simple addiction, however you're changing your whole lifestyles. Every time you cope with your frame proper, you upload every other layer of buffer (stamina) on your machine, ultimately lengthening your existence expectancy.

6. THE THREE PHASES (PHASE 3)

Phase three is if you have no starvation movements. Now, your stomach does now not crave for food love it used to months inside the past. You may revel in starvation whilst you do not eat your lunch on time, however you can cope with the put off.

First, allow me recap the stages a piece.

Phase 1: 1st month~

Phase 2: 2nd~4rd months

Phase 3: fifth Month~

Phase 1 need to be your first month. You lose weight like fast and substantially. You can cheat and it is good enough. It is a drastic alternate in lifestyles fashion except. Your body is going through fast changes. You awaken very early in the morning like 1 or 2AM within the morning. You do not recognise what to do. That is on the equal time as you start your day. You also can every now and then (like more than one times each week) consume breakfast due to the truth you wakened early out of starvation. It is the start of a modern caveman fashion life.

Your health figures enhance considerably. Especially, the liver degrees will bypass down as your food consumption goes down substantially. Your go with the flow issues will reduce. You can also drink 100-200ml duration (toddler's length juice) or have slight snacks like potato chips or 1/2 a sandwich to fight your starvation.

------------------If you stop right right here, you're losing to yoyo. Your health will skip again to in which it changed into. Actually, it is going to turn worse. That is what a yoyo does------------------------

Phase 2 is the version duration in that you keep to want to cheat every so often. You nevertheless fear and feature some doubts about the tool. However, your ldl ldl cholesterol degree must pass down until it turns regular (tons less than 200mg/dl). You although shed pounds, however no longer very an awful lot.

Your body is now very sensitive to the food that you devour. Therefore, it's far a incredible time to test what shape of meals receives you fat and what does not.

For me it modified into the Chinese meals (no offense) due to the fact I turned into ingesting too much sauce in evaluation to the Chinese. Chinese human beings consume with chopsticks and keep away from ingesting all the oily sauce. They simply dip it gently. You need to discover your horrible consuming behavior and connect them.

----------------------If you save you here, that is due to the fact you recognise you can not keep on to your vintage behavior or grasp out along side your buddies and families. However, you need to never supply in. Moreover, you can though hold out with them. You can simply do greater for them------------------

Phase three is the stabilization period in which you now not combat hunger. If you're nevertheless overweight, you may maintain to shed pounds (1-2 kilos constant with month) and your BMI (Body

Mass Index) discern will maintain to decorate (a lot much less than 25%) until you're announcing forestall. You simply comprehend that it isn't always smart to cheat, so that you do not cheat the least bit. You now not need to drink tea, juice, or water. This is the time you begin actually knowledge your body. Your body is below manage. Food isn't your precedence in life. You are not interested in meals and do not take into account food as a bargain. You most effective think about meals as quickly as an afternoon.

You are interested by your self, your work and the humans around you. You can sincerely consciousness in your lifestyles. You can be slightly obese, but you are not concerned about it. Because , you may address it. You additionally are not worried about retaining your healthful life-style. You preserve it and take out greater of the useless elements together with chocolate or others. You try to beautify your food consumption via ingesting extremely good and nutritious meals. You keep away from oily food or some other horrible food, because of the reality your frame is aware about it, and you understand it. You can not really provide an explanation for it why, however it in fact works that way.

Your belly is smaller and weaker (that means eating normal amounts) so you can not cope with the urge for meals you used to have months within the past. You attempt, however you actually can not. You wake up easy and you are prepared for a few exclusive splendid day. You enjoy less underneath the climate, due to this your aches reduce or even disappear. You are not below the have an effect on of the weather. Whether it's far wet, warm, or bloodless, you are although brilliant, healthful, and satisfied you.

Chapter 6: The Seven Principles And Dieting For Life

Now that you have professional your frame to tell the reality, listen in your body. Eat what you sense like consuming. Your body will allow you to understand what to devour. Talk on your doctor. Go to a medical institution and test your health on normal foundation.

In the vintage days, weight loss plan supposed, the manner you ate. Today, it simply means, "to shed kilos." This is the wrong belief and everybody is privy to that.

We need to offer this word its right that means once more. You can do this via the use of the usage of announcing the subsequent to yourself.

"To weight loss program way to eat and live nicely for the relaxation of my lifestyles."

People try to lose their weight in a single day when it takes months and years for them to advantage weight. Shouldn't the reverse appear slowly? I count on so and section 3 is all about this.

One answer that I placed thru this software program became that weight-reduction plan is a sequence of existence lengthy conduct. It is a lifestyle and you need to choose out the proper way to devour and stay for the relaxation of your lifestyles.

I started out out this ebook with Dr. Nagumo Yoshinori's 7 ideas.

1. Eat complete food

2. Enjoy the meals as masses as you may by way of using eating it slowly

3. Avoid caffeinated beverages or strength drinks

4. Chew gums

5. Learn to revel in fasting

6. Do not exercising excessively

7. Learn to sleep on an empty belly.

At first, training those seven ideas ingesting one meal an afternoon seemed enormously tough. But now, that's what I do ordinary. I now not drink soda, coffee, or tea. My frame is privy to they may be now not actual for me. I don't overeat, I don't exercising to lose weight (truely tone up my muscle companies.), and I sleep for at the least four, six or 8 hours.

All my stages (liver, ldl ldl ldl cholesterol, blood strain, sugar) are regular. I have no motion troubles, aches, or muscle pains. Even despite the fact that I devour chocolate and chew gums, my enamel are first-rate. I don't have any trouble going to own family dinners or formal dinners. My pals, family and I even though get along nicely notwithstanding the reality that I most effective eat lunch with them. I eat after I need to, however I don't as soon as I don't want to.

I recognize a way to combat hunger and I do it well. This on my own takes away a number of the stress that I used to have. I no longer bear in mind food tons or spend a bargain time on meals shopping for. Now I actually have more time to spend on artwork, family, and on self-improvement. What are the possibilities of my existence getting higher? Very immoderate.

This is why it's miles a leap ahead weight loss plan with health, electricity, and recognition. And it is a brief bulletproof diet.

Today, I am healthful, younger, and happy and so want to you.

Chapter 7: What Is Intermittent Fasting?

Intermittent Fasting is a form of ingesting plan in that you exchange amongst Fasting and consuming often.

Whereas many diets offer hobby to what to eat, intermittent Fasting concentrates truely on at the same time as to devour. You best devour inside the accredited hours even as you exercise intermittent Fasting.

Our our our bodies have evolved to head without consuming for hours, days, or weeks. Early people have been hunters and gatherers who evolved the ability to spend extended periods with out food earlier than studying to plant vegetation. They had no opportunity because searching video games and amassing nuts and berries required tons time and effort.

It changed into easy to preserve a healthy weight even 50 years inside the past.

There were no computer systems, and television suggests stopped human beings from consuming through manner of 11pm due to the fact they went to mattress at the same time as it ended, and servings were appreciably smaller. More human beings exercised, worked, and played exterior in general.

We stay up longer to study our favorite packages, play video games, and communicate on line now that television, the internet, and distinctive forms of amusement are reachable at some point of the clock. We spend most of the day and night time ingesting and sitting.

Consuming more energy and workout plenty plenty less can also improve the hazard of weight troubles, type 2 diabetes, coronary heart sickness, and unique illnesses; however, medical evidence suggests that intermittent Fasting may additionally moreover counter those tendencies.

Is Intermittent Fasting a fad?

People have definitely been fasting for a very long term. When there has been truely no meals available, it changed into occasionally completed out of necessity.

In different instances, it end up completed for religious motives; many faiths, in conjunction with Islam, Christianity, and Buddhism, exercise a few fasting.

When unwell, every people and specific animals regularly act instinctively. Fasting is glaringly now not unnatural, and our our bodies are perfectly able to withstanding prolonged fasts.

When we skip with out food for an prolonged time, our our bodies go through changes that permit us to live on throughout famine. Hormones, genes, and important mobile restore mechanisms are all involved.

While fasting, we revel in large drops in blood sugar and insulin stages and a sharp boom in human increase hormone.

Intermittent Fasting is a well-known weight reduction approach because of the truth it's miles a quick and easy manner to reduce power and burn fat.

Others do it to decorate their metabolic fitness, which genuinely influences numerous chance elements and health indicators.

Furthermore, there can be a few proof that intermittent Fasting can growth lifespan as successfully as calorie limit, constant with rodent studies.

Furthermore, some studies shows that it can useful resource in preventing sicknesses together with coronary heart contamination, kind 2 diabetes, most cancers, Alzheimer's illness, and others. Others honestly recognize how handy intermittent Fasting is.

It is a beneficial "life hack" that simplifies your life at the equal time as also improving your health; the a lot less food you have to devise, the much less complex your life can be.

It also saves time no longer getting prepared and cleaning meals for 3 to four food an afternoon or greater.

Among many, intermittent Fasting (IF) has been tested to be a a achievement technique for maintaining and enhancing a healthful manner of life. You can speedy to shed pounds, cleanse your frame, or for religious reasons. Much clinical research has been finished to assist the fitness advantages of Fasting. The effects are but encouraging, even though it has inside the essential been tested on animals.

History of Intermittent Fasting

Fasting isn't new; humans have fasted for severa reasons, which includes religious duties, famine, and in a unmarried day durations. The exercising of Fasting end up suggested through the Greek scientist Hippocrates of Cos and Aristotle and Plato, extraordinary influential Greek philosophers.

Fasting is practiced through many faiths, which incorporates Islam, Christianity, and Buddhism, to purify or cleanse a person's soul. Still, it basically interprets into the equal advantages that the Greek researchers have supported.

The predominant aim of modern-day intermittent Fasting is to frequently introduce fasting into your each day weight loss plan, which shows consuming typically maximum of the time and from time to time going without meals for an prolonged length.

Chapter 8: Your Brain On Intermittent Fasting

The outstanding healthy eating plan is a hotly debated hassle inside the fitness and health quarter. Others receive as actual with that excessive-carb, low-fat is the quality manner to devour, while others swear with the beneficial useful resource of low-carb, excessive-fat diets. Knowing who to accept as true with and what to take note of can be tough, with many opposing reviews.

Fortunately, consuming without enforcing extensive dietary limitations can help in weight reduction, thoughts health improvement, or perhaps lifespan.

Fasting, in assessment to fad diets, is as vintage as humanity, making it greater than a passing fad. You already fast each day; our our our bodies are designed to accomplish that. You speedy from the stop of your final meal at night time until breakfast tomorrow. Intermittent Fasting dreams to step by step amplify this window till your frame and mind begin to advantage.

Altering one's food regimen, which include intermittent Fasting, blessings the mind, promotes weight reduction, and protects towards excessive exceptional ailments. Here's how your mind responds to Intermittent Fasting.

Intermittent Fasting is terrific for preserving thoughts health. Metabolic switching boosts neuroplasticity within the thoughts and slows the getting old approach. This boosts thoughts overall performance and will boom the mind's resilience to illness and damage.

Furthermore, intermittent Fasting triggers autophagy.

Fasting also can beautify intellectual clarity and focus. Fasting has been associated with progressed moods and clearer thinking, that could help your mind-gut connection and lift your basic happiness level.

These tactics assist our mind (protein sparing, decreased contamination, autophagy, and extended B.D.N.F. Manufacturing). On the handiest hand, they lessen the damage finished to thoughts cells with the aid of, for example, modulating inflammatory reactions and disposing of waste from the mind. On the alternative hand, they promote healthy mind characteristic via way of stimulating cellular restore and helping in forming new mind cells and connections amongst them, which aids in brain conversation.

This technique is appreciably aided with the resource of B.D.N.F. Deficiencies on this protein had been related to growing older-related cognitive troubles alongside aspect dementia. As a surrender stop result of its neuroprotective impact, IF helps wholesome getting old.

After satisfactory six hours of Fasting, the body produces greater of the claimed human increase hormone (HGH). This hormone changes metabolism to prioritize using fats over protein. Proteins can therefore be specifically hired for cell restore and enhancing mind cellular characteristic.

Furthermore, HGH reduces contamination and promotes autophagy. Autophagy is a way that improves the health and durability of our cells through way of cleaning out and recycling unneeded or damaged mobile components (furthermore called "mobile junk"). IF moreover will increase the amount of a protein known as thoughts-derived neurotrophic element (B.D.N.F.). When the ones approaches are blended, they beautify how the mind operates.

7 Mind-Blowing Benefits of Intermittent Fasting for Your Brain

1. Initiates autophagy

Your mind "takes out the trash" that accumulates at some point of the day via carrying out a critical approach known as autophagy, activated by using intermittent Fasting. The thoughts plays a self-cleansing characteristic that assists in cellular removal, trash sweeping, and cleansing. This nightly cleansing fosters the arrival of extra younger, more healthy cells.

Numerous research have located a link among autophagy issues and neuropsychiatric ailments which includes schizophrenia, bipolar ailment, melancholy, and Alzheimer's.

2. Improves reminiscence

Timing your meals has been showed to decorate reminiscence. In this observe, usual typical overall performance on a spatial planning and jogging memory undertaking, as well as a working memory capability take a look at, advanced significantly after 4 weeks of intermittent Fasting. According to severa animal studies, intermittent Fasting improves memory and studying.

three. Improves mood

Intermittent Fasting improves your temper and decreases stress, anger, and anxiety. According to a 2018 have a study on weight loss strategies, intermittent Fasting end up associated with massive will increase in highbrow well being and unhappiness.

four. Reduces infection

Chronic inflammation has been associated with severa mind illnesses, which encompass melancholy, bipolar disease, obsessive-compulsive sickness (O.C.D.), schizophrenia, Alzheimer's disorder, and others. According to investigate published in Nutrition Research, intermittent Fasting decreases infection, which extensively benefits your intellectual and bodily fitness.

five. Fights Hyperglycemia

According to investigate posted in the British Journal of Nutrition, intermittent Fasting improves insulin sensitivity, which benefits inside the prevention of type 2 diabetes and excessive blood sugar ranges.

High blood sugar is related to a smaller hippocampus, the seahorse-formed a part of your temporal lobes that impacts your temper, memory, and gaining knowledge of.

According to awesome research, the superiority of tension and melancholy amongst sufferers with kind 2 diabetes is - 3 instances greater than within the fashionable populace.

6. Lowers Nighttime Blood Pressure

Intermittent Fasting decreases blood strain at the identical time as you sleep, this is wholesome on your coronary heart and mind because of the fact the whole thing correct for your coronary heart is also amazing in your mind. If you've got hypertension or prehypertension, your blood deliver to the mind is reduced. Low mind blood glide SPECT imaging scans have been used to diagnose melancholy, bipolar sickness, schizophrenia, ADD/ADHD, traumatic mind damage, substance misuse, suicidal ideation, and certainly one of a type ailments. Low blood go along with the drift is also the most not unusual mind imaging predictor of someone's hazard of getting Alzheimer's disorder.

7. Removes Excess Fat

When you fast from time to time, you burn more fats, which blessings your brain's fitness. Excess fats to your frame isn't always your friend. Obesity is volatile to thoughts fitness and has been linked to an multiplied danger of depression, bipolar ailment, panic illness, agoraphobia (worry of leaving the house), and addictions, in keeping with a growing frame of research, collectively with research published in Archives of General Psychiatry and Psychosomatic Medicine.

Consider adopting intermittent Fasting into your recurring due to the numerous blessings for mind health.

11 People who need to no longer do Intermittent Fasting

1. You have Sleeping Disorder

Getting authentic sufficient sleep each night time is essential for keeping emotional stability, maintaining cognitive function, and mending and regenerating muscle tissue after workout. Going to mattress hungry may make it greater hard for your body to relax and sleep since it maintains your thoughts alert and your body confused.

Inadequate sleep motives numerous fitness dangers as it interferes along with your body's herbal capability to get better and repair itself.

Furthermore, on the identical time as you spend a few hours with out consuming, your blood sugar degrees in reality drop, which might likely reason you to rouse in the nighttime feeling uneasy. The fast eye motion (R.E.M.) cycle, the maximum crucial sleep duration, is whilst disruptions can damage your health. This stage takes area severa times all through your sleep and is essential for maintaining information discovered at some stage inside the day. Of direction, in addition to having issues remembering matters, not getting sufficient sleep can cause more problems.

A loss of sleep can disrupt weight manipulate and jeopardize people's protection with the useful aid of decreasing their functionality to anticipate efficaciously.

2 You have an Eating Disorder.

Disordered ingesting is some of everyday eating patterns which could or may not help a evaluation of a particular eating sickness. Eating disorders are characterised as descriptive phrases in preference to an contamination. On the other hand, if they are no longer treated, unusual ingesting styles and behaviors may want to in all likelihood motive an eating contamination together with anorexia nervosa, bulimia nervosa, or binge consuming.

Anyone with a history of eating problems and eating troubles must keep away from trying intermittent Fasting.

People with this information may additionally extend a disordered pattern in reaction to any approach that encourages restrict. It's essential for all and sundry, but specifically for someone with this records, to pay attention to your body and what makes you experience right every physical and mentally. Limiting your eating window is not ideal for you if it does now not assist this.

3. You have an excessive exercising regime

Attempting to have a study intermittent Fasting while following an excessive workout regime is not an superb mixture. If you mechanically do CrossFit or are in marathon schooling, you must count on two instances before incorporating IF. To stay motivated, you typically want to eat some issue earlier than running out. It is also essential to eat some element after your exercising.

A strenuous workout will produce tiny muscle tears and burn up your glycogen stores. A recovery meal inner 1-2 hours, observed with the beneficial resource of everyday food each three-4 hours, can useful resource in refilling glycogen reserves and beautify muscle repair and renewal at some level within the day. Missing this put up-exercise meal can reason your healing to take longer and may even inhibit important muscle development and regeneration.

If you're aiming to expand muscle, taking protein at diverse instances at some point of the day is vital in area of cramming all of it into a single eating window. According to severa professionals, the body cannot successfully digest extra than 30-35 grams of protein in a single sitting. As a stop result, any greater protein taken inside the direction of the day that isn't always implemented (for example, via workout or weight lifting) is normally stored as fat in preference to muscle.

The fine manner to increase muscle is to unfold protein within the path of the day and take a protein-rich snack spherical one hour in advance than mattress. Narrowing your ingesting window to only 8 hours undermines this approach.

four. You have digestive troubles.

When gastrointestinal troubles are already difficult to address, which includes an inconsistent ingesting pattern in reality lets in to get worse the hassle. Intermittent Fasting may moreover exacerbate your symptoms and signs and symptoms when you have already were given digestive troubles (including I.B.S.).

IF might probably get worse digestive issues due to extended fasting durations. Fasting also can modify the usual strategies of the digestive device, resulting in constipation, indigestion, and bloating.

Furthermore, eating large meals—usually required for the kinds of IF that want an extended speedy—can motive gastrointestinal misery. I.B.S. Sufferers want to be careful because of the truth their digestive structures are already greater sensitive.

5 You want Focus and Concentration.

You will pay hobby considering the reality that ingesting offers you with power and nutrients. When you are hungry, all you can consider is meals, which takes your interest a ways out of your duties. Of direction, everyone reacts in a one-of-a-kind way to IF—it's miles primarily based upon on the person—but be warned that in case you're now not used to going with out meals for extended periods, it is able to to start with make it tough that permits you to hobby.

While a few take delivery of as real with intermittent Fasting gives them more energy, others may additionally revel in fatigued, no longer capable of reputation, or have terrible strength stages. This would possibly have an effect on your everyday challenge productivity. If your art work or sports activities want quite some electricity and hobby, intermittent Fasting may not fit you.

6. You are Diabetic

The very last component diabetics want is fasting to compound the numerous united statesand downs in blood sugar they already undergo during the day. This is in particular difficult for sufferers with type 1 diabetes because of the fact that they can't manufacture insulin, the hormone liable for transferring sugar from the bloodstream to one-of-a-kind frame cells together with muscle corporations, adipose (fats) tissue, or maybe your liver.

People with kind 1 diabetes normally require insulin injections to eat without getting hyperglycemia, a state of affairs wherein an excessive amount of sugar is in drift.

Never attempt intermittent Fasting without first touring a clinical health practitioner and being very well supervised if you're a diabetic and presently taking diabetes meds, specifically insulin. The combination of intermittent Fasting and diabetic capsules would likely bring about dangerously low blood sugar stages.

Avoid Intermittent Fasting if you have low blood sugar issues because of the fact you need to eat frequently to preserve your blood sugar ranges steady.

7. You are breastfeeding or pregnant.

IF involvement may additionally furthermore jeopardize a little one's development even as a girl is pregnant or breastfeeding. Calorie intake at some stage in pregnancy and nursing ought to be enough to promote the toddler's real boom and milk manufacturing. Intermittent Fasting can impair your ability to eat electricity; therefore it is not encouraged for pregnant or breastfeeding women.

If you're seeking to get pregnant, IF might not be your first-rate healthy eating plan.

Intermittent Fasting can also make a contribution to reproductive troubles with the useful resource of affecting menstruation, disrupting metabolism, and possibly inducing early menopause in girls.

eight. You are on remedy

Some tablets ought to be inquisitive about meals due to the reality, among unique topics, they could purpose nausea or dizziness. Even folks that mechanically take loads of vitamins or nutritional supplements can be stricken by IF fasting intervals. For instance, those stricken by anemia or low blood iron levels may additionally need to take one or more iron dietary nutritional dietary supplements often to help repair iron tiers. Taking iron dietary supplements with food can assist in assuaging the nausea that they're regarded to purpose. An iron supplement may be taken at any time, but what in case you're taking a remedy that ought to be considering meals and at a specific time of day? Finally, starting this eating regimen isn't a excellent idea if it does no longer paintings at the side of your medicinal drug while you take into account that this is while things become a bit sticky.

9. You have a inclined immune device.

People who have genuinely recovered from or are presently coping with a top infection ought to no longer interact in IF with out in search of authorization from a physician. Enough caloric consumption is frequently important to keep lean frame mass and a robust immune device in individuals with most cancers or weakened immune structures. Before challenge intermittent Fasting, the ones people have to see a clinical scientific physician.

10. You can not include it into your manner of lifestyles.

Your capability to engage in IF effectively is probably considerably confined via your technique time desk.

For instance, what may need to you do if one in each of your meal instances came about inside the course of the day but you had to sleep in the path of the day due to the fact you worked the night time time shift? Worse, what if the majority of your rapid takes place while you are at art work? What in case you changed shifts every day and in no way saved to a regular agenda?

Intermittent Fasting can deliver complications, temper fluctuations, and a enjoy of chilly. These capability facet results may also prevent you from on foot and reduce your productiveness.

eleven. You are not ready to exercising Intermittent Fasting.

Intermittent Fasting dreams a remarkable deal of highbrow fortitude. Going without food for prolonged periods needs plenty of electricity of mind. If you aren't emotionally organized for this, you can expand a awful relationship with food. Your fixation with food sooner or later of Fasting may also spark off you to overeat and binge in some unspecified time in the future of non-fasting durations.

Chapter 9: Pros & Cons Of Intermittent Fasting

10 Pros of Intermittent Fasting

Several studies have positioned that following an intermittent fasting everyday can assist with weight loss, reminiscence and intellectual commonplace typical overall performance improvement, cardiovascular fitness, kind 2 diabetes manipulate, and most cancers remedy efficacy.

Although most of this research is primarily based mostly on animal research, new human facts screen promising consequences, in particular in terms of the capability to assist in weight loss and enhance different factors of vitamins-related continual ailments which consist of diabetes and heart sickness.

Although the extended-time period effects of intermittent Fasting have not all started to be very well researched, new research has positioned a few encouraging short-term advantages, which we've got got highlighted right proper here. While the functionality advantages of Fasting are attractive, there may be inadequate statistics to complete that it's miles proper to a number one healthy weight loss plan for weight loss or health improvement.

1. Aids in Weight Loss

It is wellknown records that the amount of food ate up, in preference to the frequency or time of food, is a decisive element for weight loss. With intermittent Fasting, you may be capable of maintain a calorie deficit that leads to weight reduction.

Intermittent Fasting, but, does not continually imply a calorie deficit. Even with a restrictive consuming technique, a few warfare to hold a wholesome calorie variety.

Calorie restrict has been proven to lower body weight and visceral fat; however, preserving a healthy caloric deficit over lengthy periods can be tough. As recent human research suggests giant reductions in frame weight and visceral fats, intermittent Fasting is a practical weight loss approach.

Because it may be difficult to result in human beings to reduce their eating whilst nonetheless fasting, and variables which include protein intake, period of Fasting, and food exquisite may additionally moreover have an impact on consequences, intermittent Fasting is a hard intervention to check in the long run. It is uncertain whether or no longer or no longer weight loss plan or weight benefit is likely as soon as Fasting is discontinued; as a result, further study is wanted to decide any long-time period weight reduction advantages of intermittent Fasting.

Weight loss through intermittent Fasting may match past mere calorie manipulate. Fasting's physiological outcomes, which includes decreased tiers of the hormones leptin and insulin, may result in extra weight loss than calorie restrict by myself.

Finally, retaining a healthful weight dreams more than in reality regulating our calorie intake through techniques together with intermittent Fasting. Our potential to lose and keep weight depends on different factors, which consist of our way of lifestyles, strain degrees, sleep patterns, and so forth.

Weight loss may be helped by using way of way of intermittent Fasting, which may furthermore have an impact on the opposite blessings of Fasting.

2. Increases Insulin Resistance.

Intermittent Fasting and weight loss assist reduce fasting blood glucose and beautify insulin sensitivity thru manner of lowering leptin concentrations (a hormone generated via fat cells to modulate urge for food). It will also growth adiponectin concentrations (a hormone implicated in glucose and lipid metabolism).

People who fasted once in a while had lower blood glucose degrees in trials wherein Fasting emerge as used as a weight reduction intervention and method for keeping a wholesome weight, every of which can be important dreams in stopping and treating diabetes.

These capacity advantages may be stimulated extra by way of calorie limit-caused weight reduction and body fat percent reductions. However, proof suggests that intermittent Fasting has a commonly extraordinary effect on blood sugar ranges.

Intermittent Fasting can help humans with and with out diabetes shed pounds and enhance their glycemic manage and insulin resistance.

three. It May Help Lower Cholesterol

If you eat a nutritious weight loss program whilst you are not fasting, your ldl cholesterol may also moreover lower because of intermittent Fasting.

Intermittent Fasting has been connected to higher lipid profiles in healthful and obese people, along with decrease levels of everyday ldl cholesterol, LDL (low-density lipoprotein), and triglycerides.

Because the bulk of studies exploring its consequences has been accomplished on oldsters fasting for Ramadan, intermittent Fasting may be an effective dietary technique for decreasing ldl ldl ldl cholesterol. More check is wanted, however, to recognize the variations amongst short-term and lengthy-term metabolic changes because of Fasting.

If you are concerned about cholesterol levels, strive incorporating healthful lifestyle picks at the side of frequent workout and a diet plan rich in excessive-fiber, low-saturated fats food.

four. Promotes Heart Health

Intermittent Fasting may additionally additionally protect human hearts thru preventing coronary heart contamination and developing restoration after coronary coronary coronary heart assaults, regular with statistics from big animal research.

Human research have examined that intermittent Fasting can decrease threat elements associated with an accelerated danger of heart infection.

five. Lowering blood stress

Lowering ldl ldl ldl cholesterol and fats ranges within the blood, lowering inflammatory symptoms collectively with C-reactive proteins and cytokines that modify blood sugar tiers

The metabolic changes and calorie restrict related to intermittent Fasting can also lessen your resting coronary coronary heart rate (H.R.). Heart charge rises, accelerated blood waft, and vasodilation.

While this may seem interesting, human beings do not usually respond to remedy alternatives like animals do. More human have a study is needed to surely apprehend the characteristic of intermittent Fasting in coronary coronary coronary heart infection. The terrific of your vitamins is likewise especially essential in your coronary coronary coronary heart's fitness.

A food plan rich in nutrient-dense whole foods which includes entire grains, fruits, greens, and amazing meats stays the best technique for supporting coronary coronary heart fitness.

5. It May Help Reduce Inflammation

Inflammation happens actually in our our our bodies as a part of defending toward volatile micro organism or recuperation wounds by means of way of the use of activating our immune structures.

However, if infection persists for an extended duration, it could begin to damage us. Chronic infection happens at the same time as the immune device is continuously aroused with the aid of something it perspectives as a risk. Chronic infection impacts persistent health situations which encompass atherosclerosis, coronary heart illness, osteoporosis, and diabetes.

Intermittent Fasting has been demonstrated to reduce ranges of pro-inflammatory markers collectively with homocysteine, interleukin, and C-reactive protein, all of which make contributions to the improvement of many chronic ailments.

A rigorous anti-inflammatory eating regimen, the automobile-immune protocol, or anti inflammatory meals may also all help in lowering contamination within the body.

While Fasting also can have sure fitness benefits, adjusting our diet and way of lifestyles also can help us assemble healthful behavior for you to enhance our well-being.

6. Helps to maintain brain health and function.

Intermittent Fasting may additionally decorate thoughts health and characteristic thru preventing thoughts neurons from degenerating and malfunctioning. It may furthermore beautify reminiscence and highbrow ordinary performance and sell mind health.

According to a cutting-edge study, intermittent Fasting can also efficiently treat neurological sicknesses which include epilepsy, Alzheimer's, Parkinson's, and stroke.

Remember that those capability benefits can also stem from extra than without a doubt fasting; reduced contamination, decrease frame fat, and advanced blood sugar levels have all been connected to genuine mind feature.

7. Keeps cells sturdy and colourful

When we fast, we permit our our bodies to rest and repair whilst moreover looking after the incorporated systems that maintain our cells wholesome. Our our our bodies really undergo procedures like autophagy to keep our cells healthy, which keeps us healthful.

Autophagy is even as our cells discard waste and faulty cells to assist our our our our bodies cleanse diseased cells and regenerate new, extra healthful ones. Intermittent Fasting, regular with information, will growth the frequency of this system, making our structures work harder to smooth any extra waste and malfunctioning cells.

Increased autophagy also can resource in stopping severa illnesses, which include most cancers, inflammatory problems, cardiovascular infection, and neurological problems.

8. You Could Live a Longer Life

Intermittent Fasting may additionally additionally furthermore assist us live longer lives at the same time as also developing the wonderful of our lives because of various reasons, inclusive of weight reduction, decreased blood stress, and the bulk of the abovementioned benefits.

Animal studies have indicated that intermittent Fasting improves existence expectancy and the markets for pressure, health, metabolic reaction, and age-associated ailments.

Given the more than one variables that effect epidemiological research and the remarkable form of fasting behaviors, validating the ones findings in human trials is tough. However, some blessings of intermittent Fasting may also moreover ultimately beautify our traditional splendid of life and reduce our hazard of continual ailments.

9. Could Play a Role in Cancer Prevention and Treatment

This potential benefit continues to be a hint hazy. According to animal fashions, fasting frequently also can help shield regular cells from the damaging outcomes of chemotherapy capsules at the identical time as making most cancers cells extra receptive to the treatment.

The evidence for human trials remains inconclusive. However, further research is wanted to properly draw close the capability blessings of fasting in maximum cancers remedy. Losing weight and decreasing infection in the body might also additionally lessen the hazard of growing most cancers.

10. Can help within the Promotion of Balance in Sectors Other Than Food

Since we are limited to meals in the course of intermittent Fasting, it is the primary element that consists of mind. However, would a break from different factors of our lives be beneficial?

What else are we able to speedy from besides food, for the reason that the simple guideline of Fasting is to abstain from a few aspect for a very particular time?

We can gain from a harm from tv, social media, video video video video games, cellphone, and so on. This would possibly likely benefit our fitness and well-being.

Finally, consciously converting or adjusting our sports activities may also assist us boom values- and notion-based totally fitness and health dreams.

three Cons of Intermittent Fasting

Overall, certainly intermittent Fasting gives fitness advantages. Every weight loss program, but, also can have downsides if no longer followed efficiently.

The following are 4 ability dangers or "cons" of intermittent Fasting:

1. Intermittent Fasting despite the reality that reasons weight gain.

If they sense hungry during their fasting duration, some people can be extra willing to participate in binge behaviors even as not fasting. Even in case you fast for 12-16 hours every day, ingesting extra strength than your frame utilizes will result in lengthy-term fat accumulation.

In brilliant words, you hazard gaining weight if you have problem handling your hunger and bingeing at some point of your non-fasting intervals.

Going rogue throughout your non-fasting instances might also damage your efforts to shed kilos. Establish a meal schooling ordinary or plan your meals to make certain you provide your frame with what it requires.

When fasting, you might nonetheless gain weight in case you ingest extra energy than your body burns. Intermittent Fasting isn't always a alternative for correct food or calorie control.

2. Missed food may additionally reason nausea, dizziness, and headaches.

Fasting for an prolonged time may additionally additionally reason your blood sugar degrees to plummet, making you feel faint, woozy, headachey, and/or nauseated.

If you've got have been given a systematic circumstance, test collectively along with your medical physician to determine if intermittent Fasting is steady. People with type 1 diabetes who additionally use diabetic medicinal drugs can be extra prone to significant facet effects or have problem retaining blood sugar manipulate.

Consider beginning a fasting practice on a day or time on the equal time as you won't need to be significantly busy or intensely targeted because your frame will want a while to modify.

three. Restrictive Eating Can Lead to Eating Disorders

Any weight loss program emphasizing meal skipping or limited eating may additionally purpose terrible meals institutions. Particularly on the same time as limiting or skipping meals has a right away horrible effect at the advantages of weight reduction.

This is not a healthy way to approach fasting and may cause disordered consuming behavior or slipping right proper right into a vicious cycle of eating regimen for some people.

Not to mention that consuming fewer power than you need each day to satisfy your fundamental desires may result in nutrition deficiency, reduced immunity, and notable health problems.

Be absolutely honest with yourself earlier than setting out any fasting workout. You have to additionally are looking for recommendation out of your practitioner earlier of time when you consider that a aware or intuitive feeding plan may be desired.

For whichever motive you make a decision to exercise Intermittent Fasting, preserve in thoughts that simple nutrients necessities like calorie restrict and a balanced meal will allow you to be successful.

Any hopes of reaping the fitness advantages of intermittent Fasting may be destroyed in case you behave unreasonably within the direction of your non-fasting periods.

Chapter 10: The Do's And Don'ts Of Intermittent Fasting

Intermittent fasting effectiveness relies upon on how strictly you adhere to and have a look at your approach. You have to additionally be privy to some dos and don'ts whilst adopting intermittent Fasting as a weight-loss technique.

The listing of dos and don'ts below consists of important facts about intermittent Fasting.

The 5 Do's of Intermittent Fasting

Examine your frame.

Starting a quick for the entire day or some hours may be horrifying and tough. Success want to pay heed on your frame's cues. Begin cautiously, be aware about any unsightly results or symptoms of weariness, and consume some thing if you are hungry.

Eat Fibre and Fatty Foods.

Foods with prolonged fiber content fabric will keep you nourished for longer with food excessive in healthy fats.

Plan in advance of time

You should have a plan if you desire to prevail at a few element. Intermittent Fasting certainly falls internal this institution. To increase a fasting plan, you need to first define your dreams and motives for Fasting. To guarantee that your plan is adequately unique to make sure that it benefits you, you should moreover consider organic attributes precise to you, in conjunction with any present medical ailments.

Visit your medical doctor to get their recommendation before setting out any diet or intermittent fasting ordinary.

Drink severa water.

You should avoid dehydration when you recollect that you will be purposely depriving yourself of food. Water intake is crucial for the duration of an intermittent speedy.

What can I drink if I'm fasting? This is a question to which a professional nutritionist could right now reply: water.

Water makes your belly experience entire at the equal time as you fast, suppressing your starvation. On a standard day, you may drink a couple glasses of liquid, and the water in your meals keeps you hydrated. When intermittent Fasting, you stay hydrated thru eating more water to trap up at the water loss caused by the absence of food ingested.

Take care of your body.

There isn't always any way to expect how you may react to Fasting before you start it due to the reality each person's bodies react otherwise. Pay unique hobby to any adjustments on your frame, your diploma of power, or each one of a kind terrible signs that could increase as soon as you start fasting. Stop fasting as speedy as you revel in inclined, lightheaded, or now not capable of perform your each day sports activities.

When you first start fasting, you may enjoy worn-out or sluggish due to the fact your body consumes a good deal less energy than it is used to. You need to spoil your fast or are searching for clinical interest if this sensation persists.

The five Don'ts of Intermittent Fasting

Do no longer fast if you have a systematic state of affairs.

Fasting is not suitable for every person. Whether you are pregnant, have a continual illness, or are on medicine, your body calls for all the electricity it could get.

Fasting isn't recommended since it deprives the frame of this power. Although intermittent Fasting is often a manner to shed kilos and preserve it off, different weight reduction strategies may additionally additionally moreover healthy your specific desires. Speak collectively with your clinical medical health practitioner to analyze extra about the weight reduction options that may be only for you.

Limit your intake in advance than your fasting day.

If you recognize you won't be eating lots, if some thing, day after today, you will be tempted to overeat the night time earlier than. Choose nutrient-dense food such as carbohydrates, proteins, and unsaturated fats due to the reality your body needs slow-burning materials to offer you power for the following day.

When fasting, avoid doing anything that requires masses of electricity.

If you want to reduce or hold the burden you've got already misplaced, you should stability nutrients (Fasting) and pastime. Exercising or sporting out distinct strenuous sports is not encouraged whilst fasting. Light to moderate interest is advanced to strenuous exercising, in accordance to analyze.

Overdoing it could injure your body and negatively effect your highbrow fitness, making it extra difficult to paste for your fasting recurring. Simultaneously, face up to the use of your fast as an excuse to do not something except lay approximately.

Avoid Calorie Restriction

Eating time offers your body with the strength it wants to feature. While limiting your calorie intake ultimately of this era can be tempting, doing so can also additionally obstruct your improvement, make your body hungrier than normal, and compel you to break your fast in advance than you're equipped.

Do not Binge Eat after breaking your Fast.

Bingeing is the polar opposite of calorie restrict. Furthermore, you'll eat greater power, negating the blessings of fasting without a doubt.

Avoid overworking your frame.

Your frame does no longer obtain the regular electricity out of your everyday meals at the identical time as you fast. While it is appropriate to exercise as everyday, it's far vital to avoid overexerting your body.

To exercise intermittent Fasting successfully, you want to don't forget even as and what you ingest. Begin with a practical fasting-to-eating ratio, and you will supply your self a excellent hazard of achievement.

Chapter 11: Intermittent Fasting And Weight-Loss

Finding the food regimen that is the very great to study even as notwithstanding the reality that being the high-quality is DIFFICULT! There have been severa articles, internet sites, books, and special courses in this trouble. Some are scientifically based totally absolutely, whilst others, well, are not.

One weight loss plan approach that has currently won choose is Intermittent Fasting. One of the motives for its popularity is that intermittent Fasting is beneficial.

What's the Difference among Weight Loss vs. Fat Loss?

While masses folks profess to want to shed kilos, the majority human beings simply satisfactory need to lose fat. There is, clearly, a large difference.

Simply placed, weight reduction implies a lower within the range on the size. That quantity does not reflect what you have were given misplaced. Because frame fluids and muscle businesses can be misplaced similarly to weight, dropping weight is generally misleading.

Body water loss is notably commonplace. When you sweat or urinate, as an instance, you lose body water. Your weight may be affected, but it'll go lower back to normal even as you hydrate.

Many people lose muscle businesses after they bypass on a weight loss program. Because muscle tissues take a number of electricity, this circumstance is undesirable. When you lose muscle companies, your each day calorie expenditure decreases. This might also moreover moreover motive you to eat more energy than you burn over time, growing your body fats.

Losing fats includes doing precisely this: decreasing your frame fat percent. Regardless of the weight reduction technique, the motive need to be to lose fats mass.

Calorie Restriction and Fat Loss

The most commonplace weight reduction (or fats-loss) approach is calorie restriction. Unwanted side results of lengthy-time period calorie limit encompass weight loss plateaus, regaining fats whilst consuming usually another time, hormonal pathway modifications reduced bone density, and muscular tissues loss.

Weight Loss Through Intermittent Fasting

After reading approximately a number of the issues of calorie limit, you may be asking whether or not intermittent Fasting is a great technique that allows you to now not bring about any of the awful factor results we without a doubt said. The brief answer is that it maximum really has the capability to be a higher possibility!

Intermittent Fasting Improves your general fitness

To begin with, intermittent Fasting has been time and again confirmed to gain health. It can also assist to decrease contamination, insulin resistance, and the risk of cardiovascular illness.

Fasting makes you more "metabolically bendy" or "metabolically inexperienced"; consequently, it is able to be a better opportunity for fat loss than calorie restriction. What is the importance of this? When it comes to developing strength, your body uses stored fats more efficiently than stored sugar, referred to as "metabolic flexibility."

You ought to educate your body to try this. Fasting over an prolonged length (12+ hours) to set off your body to lose the bulk of its sugar shops is the quality way to train your frame (glycogen). When this takes area, your body will use its fat reserves as an power supply.

Some scientists discuss with this transition as "turning on the metabolic switch." After a few repetitions, your body turns into extra skilled at the usage of unique metabolic pathways to burn fat for electricity—mechanisms it could now not rent frequently. You grow to be greater metabolically adaptable at the same time as your frame has been skilled to use more fats inside the path of the day.

When you suggest your body to burn more stored fat for electricity, you are essentially telling it to use your fat shops. This method that no matter what you do— searching T.V., walking, taking walks, and so on.—your body will burn more fats for electricity.

People which may be greater metabolically bendy have a propensity to have decrease body fat opportunities and are leaner. Furthermore, metabolic flexibility seems to be a few component your frame can keep over the years; consequently, if you prevent intermittent Fasting, it's going to no longer just vanish.

According to studies, boosting your frame's metabolic flexibility advantages weight loss. It decreases your chance of getting high great issues.

According to experts, this explains why you could no longer lose muscle businesses while fasting. Furthermore, your muscle tissue preserve fat, which they may use as energy in case you exercising or flow about. If your frame isn't always nicely-professional to apply fats as a gasoline supply, it is able to and will damage down your muscle groups for strength.

Intermittent Fasting boosts boom hormones

Another element that can save you your frame from losing muscular tissues is that human growth hormone degrees upward push even as you rapid. This hormone additionally boosts fats burning on the identical time as protecting muscle groups for your body.

Finally, fats loss is distinct from weight reduction. When beginning a brand new food plan, the goal need to be to shed fats at the same time as preserving muscles.

Chapter 12: Types Of Intermittent Fasting

It's terrific that there are such some of precise methods to exercising IF. If you're interested by doing so, you could choose out the approach that extraordinary suits your manner of life, boosting your possibilities of success.

7 Types of Intermittent Fasting

Here are the seven sorts of Intermittent Fasting

1. The 5:2 Plan

This is one of the maximum well-known IF techniques. Eat usually for five days (do not be counted power) and then consume 500 or 600 power each day for women and men at the final days. Fasting days is probably any day of the week which you choose.

Short fasting instances are designed to keep you cooperative; in case you are hungry on a fasting day, honestly consider the following day on the equal time as you may "dinner party" yet again. For some people, a 5:2 weight-reduction plan may be more a achievement than a calorie restriction for the entire week.

Avoid fasting on days at the same time as you will be doing strenuous patience exercising. If you are getting prepared for a cycling or taking walks race (or making plans immoderate-mileage weeks), bear in thoughts if this form of Fasting will artwork into your schooling program. Consult a sports activities activities nutritionist as a substitute.

2. Time-limited Fasting

This type of IF consists of deciding on a every day consuming window that, ideally, leaves a 14- to 16-hour fasting window.

This technique permits you to pick out out your ingesting window from nine am to five pm. It may be specifically excessive best for a person with a circle of relatives who already eats a past due meal. The relaxation of the time spent fasting is spent sleeping. You do not want to miss any food relying on at the same time as you place your window. However, how everyday you're will decide this. Daily Fasting may not be for you if your time table is unpredictable and also you require or select the freedom to go out for breakfast, pass on a overdue date, or attend glad hour often.

3. Overnight Fasting.

This method, the simplest of the types available, consists of fasting for 12 hours every day. For example, prevent ingesting after supper at 7 pm and resume eating breakfast day after today at 7 am. Autophagy remains operating at 12 hours, but the cell benefits are a whole lot much

much less vast. This is the essential minimal of fasting hours.

This approach is useful because of its simplicity. Furthermore, you aren't missing meals; you're foregoing a night time snack (in case you ate one, initially). This method, however, falls quick of optimizing the benefits of Fasting. If you are using Fasting to shed pounds, a narrower fasting window provides you extra time to eat, which might not assist you decrease your calorie intake.

four. Eat Stop Eat

This fasting method differs from others in that you location a top magnificence on flexibility. The idea is that Fasting is merely a brief wreck from eating. You commit to a resistance exercise time table and one or 24-hour fasts weekly. When your speedy is over, generally consume and act as even though nothing passed off. I'm completed now. Nothing else.

To eat as it should be, you have to return to a regular ingesting time table. This includes not bingeing after a short, abstaining from excessive diets, and ingesting a great deal less than required. The outstanding fats-loss plan mixes normal weight education with unusual Fasting. Allowing yourself one or 24-hour fasts in some unspecified time inside the destiny of the week will assist you to devour a piece more on the very last 5 or six non-fasting days. As a end result, he gives, concluding the week with a calorie deficit without feeling obligated to conform with a rigorous food plan is an awful lot much less hard and extra a laugh.

five. One Meal A Day

Here, you surely devour as fast as a day. This technique approach consuming dinner after which forgoing meals until day after today's dinner. Unlike 5:2, while the fasting period is 36 hours, complete-day Fasting calls for fasting from dinner to dinner or lunch to lunch. For instance, you may have supper on Sunday, then 500-six hundred electricity on Monday to "speedy," discovered thru breakfast on Tuesday.

The advantage of fasting one meal an afternoon for weight loss is that consuming all the electricity for the day right now's difficult but now not now not possible. The downside of this method is that it is hard to get all of the vitamins your frame dreams in a unmarried meal to function properly.

Not to mention that sticking to this approach may be difficult. You may be so hungry via dinner that you pick out horrible, calorie-dense meal options. Consider this: Broccoli isn't exactly what you need to consume while you're hungry. For example, many people overindulge in espresso to avoid starvation, which may negatively effect their functionality to sleep. You also can enjoy cognitive fog at a few degree within the day if you do no longer consume.

6. Alternate-Day Fasting

On days after they do no longer rapid, people may additionally choose to consume best 25% of their every day caloric consumption (or form of 500 energy). This technique to weight loss is famous. Fasting on trade days has been discovered in research to significantly lessen frame mass index, weight, fats mass, and ordinary ldl ldl cholesterol in overweight patients.

You can be involved that you can't be fulfilled in case you rapid. The hunger-related terrible results of exchange-day

Fasting commenced to fade via week and enhance via week 4. The disadvantage of this manner is that it can be difficult to implement because of the truth check humans said that they were in no way actually "whole" for the duration of the 8-week check.

7. Choose Your Fasting Day

This type of IF is greater like deciding on your very personal adventure. Practice time-restricted fasting each specific day or a couple of instances every week (for example, fast for 16 hours and eat for eight). This way that Sunday can be a normal eating day, with you finishing at 8 pm and starting once more at midday on Monday. In essence, it is similar to once in a while skipping breakfast.

Remember that there may be contradictory statistics approximately the impact of skipping breakfast on weight loss. No convincing records enables the idea that skipping breakfast influences weight. However, several research have decided that having breakfast has little effect on weight reduction. Furthermore, some studies have related skipping breakfast to an improved chance of demise from cardiovascular sickness.

This method can be greater adaptable and fluid, allowing you to make it paintings even if your schedule varies from week to week. However, a more comfortable technique might also additionally additionally bring about softer advantages.

Chapter 13: One Meal A Day O.M.A.D

One Meal a Day (or O.M.A.D.) is one of the many kinds of intermittent Fasting. Many people will inform you without delay that O.M.A.D. Is an ingesting disorder, but that is simplest due to the fact we've got were given been conditioned to accept as true with that ingesting 3 meals and snacks every day is the healthiest consuming sample.

No clinical proof enables the notion that eating three meals every day is the healthiest meal plan. Several research have determined that eating fewer meals day by day can assist with weight reduction and particular additives of general health.

What is O.M.A.D.?

O.M.A.D. Is one of the greater "immoderate" types of intermittent Fasting because all energy should be ingested internal one to 2 hours. If you want to stick to this food regimen efficiently, you need to furthermore make the effort to be steady with whilst making a decision to eat.

In specific phrases, you consume at the same time each day. Some human beings may additionally moreover have a hearty breakfast once they upward push up and then rapid for the the rest of the day, on the equal time as others may moreover pick to fast all day and eat later in the nighttime.

You moreover need to be extremely careful about getting sufficient energy. Food is designed to feed the frame, and depriving it of gas for an extended duration can damage your health.

It is typically understood that ingesting too few electricity could have terrible health outcomes which includes hormone disturbances, reduced bone density, impaired immunity, persistent weariness, and extra. This is actual no matter the reality that the idea of consuming too few energy in share to how an lousy lot you burn has been explored completely in athletes.

Furthermore, at the equal time as you become acclimated to receiving a whole lot a good deal less power, your frame modifies severa physical functions to maintain weight. In wonderful terms, your body actively opposes losing weight.

If you attempt the O.M.A.D. Eating regimen, you need to make certain you're ingesting enough power to gas your frame. Your body may additionally require a while to regulate to this new eating sample, so ingesting about 2000 power in a unmarried meal may be difficult. In evaluation, those who study the O.M.A.D. Food plan declare that your body adjusts with time, and you may have one immoderate-calorie meal.

Pros of O.M.A.D.

This approach does no longer require you to limit your calorie intake. Most diets require dieters to restriction their calorie intake. When making use of O.M.A.D., you do now not want to restrict your calorie intake. You can also consume too few energy, this is the inverse trouble. Try maintaining music of your caloric intake for a few days to make sure you get sufficient electricity for your gender, pinnacle, weight, and hobby diploma. You might also estimate your calorie intake the use of one of the severa on line applications.

By significantly prolonging your fast, you can gain all the health benefits of intermittent Fasting, together with weight loss, reduced D.N.A. Harm, anti-growing old results, and enhancements in various illness chance factors. You'll probably word outcomes right away, motivating you to maintain going.

Cons of O.M.A.D

You can also first sense surprisingly hungry. Your frame will want to alter to this sort of strict diet; therefore, there can be a learning curve. Remember that this want to simplest final a few weeks and is a brief trouble. Sipping tea and water may additionally assist you shed pounds. You need to eat some thing if you feel dizzy, queasy, or lightheaded.

O.M.A.D. Has a big capability drawback in terms of sustainability. Can you virtually maintain on with this healthy eating plan in the long run? This is truely a few issue to take into account while choosing the ideal nutritional plan. Try out some specific intermittent fasting kinds to determine which fits superb. There isn't any wrong solution.

The majority of humans regularly consume throughout the day, which can be unstable to their fitness.

You might be able to acquire some of your health-related goals by way of walking inside the direction of intermittent Fasting, along with O.M.A.D. When completed successfully, O.M.A.D. Can be a milder model of intermittent Fasting that makes you happier and extra healthy. If you have had been given any issues about O.M.A.D., you must consult your scientific health practitioner about this dietary pattern.

Chapter 14: O.M.A.D. And Weightloss

There is not any specific time to eat in the course of O.M.A.D. Fasting; some humans pick to have their one meal spherical supper, whilst others opt to devour breakfast or midday. Eating after your busiest a part of the day is generally endorsed. During Fasting, you can fulfill your urge for food by way of the usage of eating sugar-loose espresso, tea, water, or, in some times, fruit.

People at the O.M.A.D. Rapid want to encompass wholesome food to meet the body's nutritional wishes in only one hour of the day. A healthy food regimen often has hundreds of grains, beans, culmination, and vegetables.

Whether fasting or no longer, keep away from white bread, short food together with pizza and burgers, drinks, chips, and processed gadgets baked in sugar.

This intermittent fasting type has no calorie limit because of the reality the time constraint restricts how loads you may ingest. Those who preference to lose weight attempt to adopt a low-calorie, ketogenic, or low-carb healthy eating plan inside the course of the ingesting window.

According to as a minimum one have a have a have a look at, proscribing or eating an excessive amount of power at the same time as consuming reduces the advantages of intermittent Fasting; consequently, maintaining an energy stability is vital.

Is there any chance within the O.M.A.D. Eating regimen?

The dangers related with O.M.A.D. Are awesome. As a end result, you need to anticipate two times approximately the usage of it to reduce weight.

Intestinal problems:

You may additionally have bloating and digestive pain in case you overeat meals too quick. You may additionally moreover on occasion battle to eat sufficient meals to meet your calorie necessities or have constipation.

Nutritional deficiencies:

The body won't get preserve of sufficient electricity or the vital nutrients, minerals, and proteins. It can motive muscle loss, fatigue, contamination, and nutritional inadequacies.

Low blood sugar degrees - People with Type 2 diabetes who're already using blood glucose-reducing drug treatments can also moreover go through hypoglycemia because of intermittent Fasting. It can also purpose tension, wooziness, pallor, sweating, or weariness.

According to at the least one look at, missing meals will increase your hazard of immoderate blood stress and additional LDL (low-density lipoprotein), or terrible ldl ldl ldl cholesterol, for your frame. Kidney or unique cardiac issues, strokes, or excessive blood stress are all opportunities.

When the O.M.A.D. Food plan isn't always strictly accompanied, it may occasionally bring about binge consuming problems. People who abandon this approach may also moreover eat pretty some food quick because of their ongoing perception of anorexia. Ghrelin, or the hunger hormone, may additionally moreover upward thrust due to the prolonged fasting phase.

The dangers of O.M.A.D. Fasting may be mitigated through unique meal education.

O.M.A.D. Diet for Weight Loss

The O.M.A.D., like most forms of intermittent Fasting, is predicated on a calorie deficit. There isn't any hard proof that O.M.A.D. Fasting is better than other calorie-limit eating regimen regimens.

Calorie restriction and masses much less restrictive varieties of intermittent Fasting may additionally update O.M.A.D. With its guide, you could despite the fact that shed kilos and mitigate the harmful consequences of this excessive kind of Intermittent Fasting.

Many people driven to shed pounds have benefitted from the O.M.A.D. Diet and achieved outstanding results in simplest a month or maybe each week.

When fasting, electrolyte imbalance reasons complications together with complications. To preserve electrolyte balance, mixture salt and water and drink. Keeping a hectic habitual is important to hold meals from entering into the thoughts.

Discipline is wanted to avoid binge eating at the same time as at the O.M.A.D. Weight-discount plan. Long-term O.M.A.D. Dieters also record advanced cognitive feature and popularity.

Chapter 15: What Is Fasting And Why Is It Authentic For You?

Fasting is known as deliberately desisting from ingesting for numerous lengths of time. You need to be aware that the sensation of starving isn't hunger, it's far in truth the frame's way of burning stored strength. The common sense is quite easy. When the brief consumption of meals is stopped, the structures of the frame take a destroy from all of the difficult work that comes with digestion. All that more energy offers the body threat to heal and repair itself, energy moreover burn inside the system, which helps cast off toxic materials saved inside the body. Clearly, there can be not some thing 'unnatural' approximately fasting, our our our bodies are very plenty acquainted with the method and capable of deal with extended durations of not ingesting. When we rapid we get sizeable discounts in blood sugar and insulin levels, in addition to a drastic boom in human growth hormone.

When you devour much less than you need to and also you lose weight, your frame is going into starvation mode. In distinctive to shop electricity, metabolism slows down. When you are finished fasting and skip once more on your fashionable diet regime, you can regain the weight you lost. Your frame adjusts to fasting right away, so while you forestall fasting, you could experience less hungry on the start, however with time your appetite revs lower once more up. You may enjoy hungrier and be much more likely to overeat. Fasting every on occasion has superb effects, it helps you shed pounds but not for lengthy.

It is literally an powerful existence hack that might make your existence easier, at the same time as on the equal time enhancing your health. The fewer the food you intend and pay for, the less difficult your existence.

Why is it correct for you?

There are numerous blessings that encompass fasting. You should advantage from fasting bodily, mentally, and moreover fitness-practical. Everyone has a specific cause for fasting, whether you've got been endorsed to do it thru way of someone otherwise you simply sense like it is what you need at this factor, preserve within the back of your thoughts that fasting is ideal for you. It is continuously a win-win state of affairs.

Regaining insulin sensitivity

Fasting has proved to be a completely effective way of maintaining our body touchy to insulin. Most instances, even as our our our our bodies get too many carbohydrates and sugar, it may come to be insulin resistant. When the frame receives insulin resistant, ailments like type 2 diabetes begin to creep in. If you want to avoid this, it's miles very essential to hold your frame insulin-touchy, and fasting is an clean manner to obtain this.

A observe has demonstrated that intermittent fasting in adults with type 2 diabetes improved key markers for them along side their glucose stage and frame weight. If you discover yourself suffering with insulin sensitivity or diabetes, intermittent fasting ought to are available in accessible for you in normalizing topics.

Disease prevention

Experts have found that intermittent fasting prevents severa conditions and moreover illnesses. For example:

- Cancer

- Type 2 diabetes

- Heart situations

- Neurodegenerative ailments.

Secretion of HGH

HGH is the Human Growth Hormone really secreted inside the frame. The HGH stays energetic in the body superb for a few minutes. When you rapid, the secretion of the Human Growth Hormone is promoted. The secretion skyrockets, developing to as masses as 5-fold. It has been used effectively to build body mass, address weight troubles, and boom muscle strength. With the intermittent fasting, you sincerely flip your body into an powerful fats-burning tool.

Good on your brain

The mind and the bodywork hand in hand, therefore, some aspect is proper for the body is also accurate for the thoughts. In the approach of fasting, severa metabolic features stated to be vital for mind fitness are advanced. Including reduced oxidative strain, reduced infection, and reduce price in blood sugar tiers and insulin resistance, all of which come collectively for the well functioning of your thoughts.

It moreover reduces the stages of BDNF, that could be a deficiency that has been implicated in despair and severa brilliant mind troubles. Basically, what this shows is that intermittent fasting will boom the boom of recent neurons and stops the brain from harm.

Weight loss

In all honesty, plenty humans are wearing out intermittent fasting due to the reality we understand one manner or the opposite we're going to lose some greater kilos. Well, you're right because of the reality fasting will make you consume fewer meals except you are making up for it and eat extra inside the course of these few meals, you are taking in fewer calories. The breakdown of body fats is elevated on the same time as the insulin degree is diminished, hormone boom is higher, there can be an prolonged quantity of norepinephrine (noradrenaline). It motives their use to be facilitated for power. Simply positioned, intermittent fasting works every strategies, it balances the calorie equation such that it boosts your metabolic charge and at the equal time, reduces the quantity of food you consume. All in all, intermittent fasting can be taken into consideration an exceptionally effective weight reduction tool. It is likewise a completely green way of losing stomach fat.

Beneficial for coronary heart health

Currently, coronary heart contamination is the arena's largest killer. Various health markers and health hazard factors are related to each an improved or reduced threat of coronary coronary coronary heart sickness. Intermittent fasting has tested to put off awesome threat factors, along side blood strain, ordinary and LDL ldl cholesterol, blood triglycerides, inflammatory markers, and blood sugar tiers.

Extend your lifespan

This is a completely exciting advantage as it has the capacity to increase one's lifespan. Given a number of these diagnosed benefits for metabolism and the numerous fitness markers, it quality makes experience that intermittent fasting would possibly assist you stay longer and extra healthful. It might also additionally appear sort of a ways fetched, but severa research have proven that fasting can surely help you stay longer. As you become older, your frame's metabolism starts offevolved offevolved slowing down, fortunately, fasting permits accelerate your metabolism stopping lack of muscle tissue. Fasting additionally stimulates the discharge of boom hormones, leading to stepped forward bone electricity, better protein synthesis, and prolonged muscle groups. All these consequences pace down the getting older technique every internally and externally.

Promotes detoxing

Many of the meals we devour in recent times are processed and consist of a number of components, some of which is probably toxic to our our bodies. As we eat this food, we devour those pollution with them and they get stored in fat deposits across the frame. During the machine of fasting, your thoughts starts offevolved offevolved contemplating how it's going to provide the body with energy inside the absence of food, and to make certain that metabolism maintains on foot, the brain triggers the conversion of glycogen stored in the liver into strength and at the same time as that runs out, the fat deposits are burnt to offer electricity in the absence of food. As the fat deposits are burnt off to provide strength, the pollution stored inside the fats are released. These pollution are then removed from the body with the help of the liver, kidneys, and different organs, leaving your frame freed from gathered pollution.

Chapter 16: Different Kinds Of Intermittent Fasting

There are numerous particular strategies to effectively approach the intermittent fasting. However, ultimately, it all comes all the way right down to your non-public preference. You need to be prepared to discover what works for you in case you want to offer intermittent fasting a try. We all have unique our our bodies and reply in a one of a type way to effective subjects, with intermittent fasting, get equipped for a few "trial and errors".

For some people, fasting for 16 hours is a chunk of cake, at the identical time as others might probably have a tough time with it. However, those are the 4 maximum vital types of intermittent fasting:

The 24 hours rapid

This method consists of ingesting as soon as a day. Often instances, it's far completed two times-three instances in step with week. On the instances you've got got got set aside on your rapid, you need to have in mind which you are fasting completely for a full 24 hours. Most humans select out dinner-dinner or lunch-lunch due to the fact the case can be, i.E. You pick out out to consume dinner after which no longer consume another time till the following day's dinner. If your intention for IF is weight reduction, an advantage of the 24 hour speedy is that it's far maximum not likely that you'll eat an entire day's absolutely genuinely well worth of calories in nice one meal. However, you should moreover comprehend that this plan is quite hard to maintain to, as you'll likely have grow to be simply hungry by the point dinner rolls thru the use of and that would motive you to pick ingredients that are heavy on strength, no person exactly craves carrots and vegetables while they will be famished. To keep away from those, you will likely need to:

• Distract your self at some level within the day

• Include veggies on your food regimen on days whilst you are not fasting, so your frame receives used to it

• Don't laze spherical; you're more likely to interrupt your speedy even as you are bored.

• Go once more in your ordinary food regimen in your non-fasting days

• Give it area, don't pass for a 24 hour rapid 3 days in a row

The Twice a Week rapid

This limits how frequently you devour and now not what you devour, as different diets propose. It specializes in reducing your electricity at 500 for 2 days every week. During your fasting days, you want to eat extra fiber and high-protein substances, this helps fill you up while maintaining your electricity at a low degree. This very bendy and strain-free such that you may determine to pick a few element days of the week you're most busy, distracted enough to now not feel hungry. You additionally don't should rely calories or limit yourself out of your favored meals. However, for your non-fasting days, you could additionally want to comprise the addiction of reducing portions as a way to get effective fasting outcomes. With the two times every week rapid, on the identical time as you can choose any days of the week you deem in shape, keep in mind to place at least one non-fasting day in amongst them.

Time-restrained rapid

For this, there can be the sixteen/8 or 14/10. This is the way it works. For the 24 hours in a day, you positioned fasting and eating home domestic windows, so your ingesting is restricted advantageous hours of every day. For example, if you choose out the 16/8 frame, your consuming length is for eight hours and your fasting duration is probably sixteen hours. Your time frame may be from 12 am to eight pm. This method is well-known due to the fact we already rapid at the same time as we're asleep and with this method, your fasting period might increase in a single day. You can pick to copy this technique of intermittent fasting as regularly as you want. It all comes down to some thing your personal preference is in the end. For example, if you are the type to evoke yearning breakfast, this technique is probably not for you. This approach is greater of a more stable bet if you are attempting intermittent fasting for the number one time.

Alternate day fasting

This is a very smooth way to go about intermittent fasting. With the trade day fasting, for your fasting days you limit your consumption of energy. You can put quite various on it, say 500 energy constant with day or simply reduce your conventional consumption to about 25% for your non-fasting days, you resume your normal, healthy eating regimen. If you make a decision to be strict with yourself, to your fasting days you can decide to cancel calories common, i.E. 0 calorie intake.

The intermittent fasting is however no longer restricted to just 4 maximum crucial sorts. Here are a few few others:

The warrior healthy eating plan

The warrior diet plan dates another time to and of path, receives in name from the historical warriors like Spartans and Romans. They would possibly live bodily lively sooner or later of the day and eat usually in the midnight. If you pick out out the warrior weight loss plan, you speedy for approximately 20 hours, interact in a brief drastically extreme exercise, and location your eating duration in the last hours of the day. Typically, you will have both small food with a destroy in among or one unmarried large night meal.

A meal consistent with day

For this, the fasting period can be for about 21-23 hours. You place your eating length inside a 1-2 hour time-frame. This plan is not so hard to paste to because of the fact you continue to experience as complete and happy at the same time as regardless of the truth that staying on a calorie deficit. The one meal consistent with day plan is remarkable for losing fat however the fact that a totally sluggish gadget.

36 hour speedy

This can be very just like the 24 hours speedy but is prolonged simply so it has three days involved. On the primary day you get to have dinner, you speedy sooner or later of the second day then devour breakfast on day 3. This may be completed for as little or as regularly as as quickly as consistent with week, month, or 365 days.

Choose-your-day fast

This leans more inside the route of a pass-with-the-waft kind of journey. Technically, it includes randomly skipping food for the duration of the week anyways you deem suit. You can also determine now not to devour both breakfast lunch or dinner. It may be very easy to evolve to this format as it's far very flexible and might fit it in together with your manner of lifestyles without trouble. It though works with very tight schedules. Keep in mind, but, that milder approaches may moreover propose slower outcomes.

Chapter 17: Intermittent Fasting And The Keto Diet

Intermittent fasting and the keto healthy eating plan are of the freshest developments within the global proper now. Many use those techniques to control weight reduction, while many others use it to control first-rate fitness conditions. While they're both very similar, they're additionally very unique. While they may be each very popularly diagnosed for their very powerful effects, people often surprise which ones is better. The technique of keto dieting is known as ketosis. With ketosis, your frame is based on fat for gasoline and in the machine produces ketones which might be popularly stated for its health blessings. While at the keto weight loss program. You devour fewer carbohydrates, you keep mild protein consumption and your fats intake will in all likelihood increase. The cut price in the intake of carbohydrates is what places your frame within the metabolic country, ketosis. A vital difference among the keto weight loss plan and intermittent fasting is at the equal time because the keto healthy dietweight-reduction plan tells you what to consume, the intermittent fasting tells you whilst to consume it. People have questions on the keto diet plan and intermittent fasting all the time. Varying from questions like need to we integrate the 2? Which considered considered one of them is better? To questions like; which one works faster? Can I trade among every of them? Well, here are the answers to some of your questions:

Can you integrate intermittent fasting with the keto food plan?

The answer to this question is commonly inconclusive. Can you integrate the keto weight loss plan and intermittent fasting? It depends. Should you combine the keto eating regimen with intermittent fasting? Maybe. The reason for that is whilst this combination might be secure for some, it could no longer be for others. However, you want to apprehend pregnant or breastfeeding ladies and those with a information of disordered eating must keep away from intermittent fasting and the keto weight-reduction plan. Also, people with fine fitness situations, together with diabetes or coronary coronary coronary heart illness, want to speak about with a doctor earlier than combining the intermittent fasting with the keto eating regimen. While the mixture of these two has proved beneficial, it's far very important to word that it might not art work for anyone. Some may additionally enjoy negative reactions, like overeating on non-fasting days, irritability, and fatigue. They may additionally find out it extremely difficult. While this aggregate has confirmed very effective for some, it isn't essential to combine each. You are however unfastened to test and be aware what works amazing for you. But like every specific number one motion, it is useful to speak with your fitness care employer first.

Which is better?

Both of those diets could probably assist you obtain the purpose, you shouldn't definitely hotel to the possibility one while you experience like one isn't strolling for you. There might be something you're doing incorrect, the key's to make certain the diet you made a decision to go together with is properly balanced and properly planned so that you can get effective consequences. While the answer to the final question remains inconclusive, you need to recognize that training intermittent fasting is sincerely less difficult. Reason being that you may effects comply with through with intermittent fasting for an prolonged time body and now not lose muscle groups. Your metabolism will not lower as with intermittent fasting, you are not restricted to devour excellent meals which is probably excessive in fat, now not just like the keto healthy eating plan. At the same time, deciding on a plan isn't always a one-length-fits-all enjoy. Some can not fat for a long term and will probably quit intermittent fasting as fast as you get into it, so you may go with a keto diet.

How to Intermittent Fast on Keto

At this aspect, you're in all likelihood questioning how can I do keto and intermittent fasting? If you observe thru with the following few steps, it'd come without difficulty.

Pick a protocol and stick with it

When it includes fasting or locating a diet plan, they are severa protocols making it smooth to discover a method that works for you. Getting commenced, you without a doubt pick out out one of the awesome styles of intermittent fasting that there are. You should locate one which suits into your time table and every day normal to make matters art work much less difficult for you. You may also determine to go together with the change-day fasting, 16/8 fasting, five:2 food plan, or the 23/1 intermittent fasting keto.

Calculate

After deciding on the protocol you determined is extremely good for you, the following step is to get into calculating your keto macros. You must start planning out your weight loss program to your fasting days. While on the keto diet, 75 percent of full-size electricity ought to come from fat, 20 percent want to return from protein, and five percentage need to come from carbs. There numerous on-line calculators that can help decide your preferred each day calorie consumption primarily based on elements like your age, gender, and diploma of interest.

Formulate a meal plan

Once you're achieved calculating your each day vitamins and picked a protocol that works for you, you must then waft immediately to making plans out your food to get began out with the keto weight-reduction plan and intermittent fasting. Include to your meals some of wholesome fats like coconut oils, avocados, olive oil, ghee, and grass-fed butter similarly to the ideal quantity of protein food like unfastened-range chook, grass-fed meat, fatty fish, and eggs. To spice it up, you would probably need to function a few non-starchy veggies, smooth herbs, nuts, seeds, and wholesome beverages like water, bone broth, and green tea may be cherished as well.

Get to it!

At this problem, you are absolutely prepared! Don't permit every body will let you apprehend otherwise. It is now time for intermittent fasting and keto. Aside from all which you have prepare inside the preceding steps, you need to additionally stay hydrated, plan your workout intervals, and your fasting schedules. It may be very important to concentrate for your frame for the duration of this method and not push too difficult. On a vast keto eating regimen, it takes spherical 2-three days to attain ketosis but the 'intermittent fasting keto' the system may be improved because it allows your frame burn via glycogen stores to help enter ketosis.

It is dubious the fitness benefits of the combination of the fitness benefits of the keto weight loss plan and the intermittent fasting however, but it's far clean that ketone levels increase on the equal time because the plans are mixed. It can also moreover help accelerate weight loss however ultimately, all and sundry awesome and we reply in a completely unique manner to things, so this may now not artwork for all of us.

Chapter 18: Principles Of Intermittent Fasting

We in fact can't talk approximately intermittent fasting and bypass over the requirements. These are some of the assets you have to understand earlier than you delve into the arena of intermittent fasting:

Calories

In the arena of Intermittent fasting, calories rely. The intermittent fasting plan reasons weight loss by proscribing the variety of energy you eat. As the plan does no longer restrict you to positive meals and you're loose to eat a few factor you need at any time, you'll naturally decrease your calorie intake. However, if you at any point revel in like you're under-consuming and also you want to reinforce your consumption, make certain to get enough.

Eat healthily

As plenty as energy depend on this plan, you want to apprehend that macro-vitamins moreover depend. While the intermittent fasting permits you to devour something you need, you ought to recognition on excessive-nutrient meals and avoid prepackaged excessive-carb junk meals. No count how bendy the plan you have got chosen, you still need to eat sufficient vitamins to be healthful. Calories aren't all that subjects. You need to make sure that your frame is getting sufficient carbohydrates, protein, and fats just so your frame is capable of repair itself and receives fueled nicely.

Pay interest

While at the intermittent fasting plan, you want that allows you to be aware of all the small information. Remember that the reason you're at the plan within the first area is to heal your frame one manner or the opportunity. Even while ill, your body doesn't take enough meals as it generally could. This allows the body to pay attention on restoration itself and placing all of the previously stored vitamins and fat to use. Intermittent fasting is a manner of giving your frame a relaxation so it could focus on rebuilding, regenerating, and recovery itself.

End snacking

One massive rule of the intermittent fasting is NO SNACKING! When you don't snack, your stomach gets empty, your digestion is going to be a whole lot greater advanced and subsequently, you may surrender the everyday hunger and coffee energy attacks that you have now. Know that your body has been built to conform to any state of affairs it's miles in so, in a few days, you'll be nice.

Embrace hunger

This all just comes once more to emphasise the previous rule. While you may feeling hunger on this as you may on a few special plan, your body will come spherical and sooner or later get familiar with it. After more than one weeks, you want to no longer revel in as masses starvation. During the intermittent fast, starvation is a extremely good aspect.

Chapter 19: Step Thru The Use Of Step Intermittent Fasting

Here are subjects to recognize in advance than you dedicate your self to the plan and begin fasting:

• Book an appointment and talk collectively in conjunction with your clinical health practitioner earlier than you start – This facilitates immensely as it will decide how fit you are to perform the intermittent fasting, in particular in case you are already located on any medicine or have any underlying scientific situation. It is also essential to don't forget to prevent even as and in case you experience ill.

• Don't pressure it, keep it easy – Keeping it easy enables you increase steam and consistency instead of burning out proper away. Start with consuming simplest plain water, unsweetened tea, black coffee, or flat or carbonated water. Avoid burning yourself out early in the sport.

• Keep the feeding easy – Don't begin taking area diet plan sooner or later of your ordinary consuming window as an possibility keep on with your big meals.

• Set a simple time – Setting a smooth time that you may have a look at is likewise key. The set time may be adjusted in a while in line with your agenda but it will likely be smooth enough that lets in you to look at.

• Choose your days – Choosing the weekdays in preference to the weekends gives you fewer variables and additional form in your intermittent fasting. Look out for days that point passes through so speedy that you overlook to devour.

• Embrace slip-ups – Slip-americaare suitable, so on every occasion you're making or have one, forgive your self and pass on. Once a slip up occurs, there are 3 options to pick out from; start once more from day one, pick up from in which you slipped, or neglect absolutely about intermittent fasting. Out of the three alternatives, the final one need to in no manner skip your mind. So, if you ever slip up, make a desire to each choose up from in which you slipped up or start afresh from day one.

The subsequent aspect to do in the end of these is to transport in for the kill. Zero in at the primary motive you started out it. Whatever you start, be it intermittent fasting or reason getting, you want to ensure that there's some problem in it for you. What are you attempting out intermittent fasting?

•   Is it to shed kilos or to preserve weight? It doesn't constantly ought to do with losing weight, every so often, it may simply be about preserving your gift weight under take a look at and balance, so that it does no longer exceed or reduce. Intermittent fasting will growth hormones along side HGH and norepinephrine and reduces others together with insulin to make your frame burn out stored frame fats on the manner to, in turn, assist you lose fat.

•   Is it to relieve signs and symptoms with out the use of medication?

Intermittent fasting has been acknowledged to save you coronary coronary coronary heart illnesses, reduce infection, and decrease diabetes.

• Is it to prevent critical illnesses and growth your lifespan? According to research, wearing out intermittent fasting may additionally additionally moreover boom your frame's immune machine and supply the immune a lift to prevent ailments which include cancer and Alzheimer's, as well as growth your longevity.

You may additionally even need to address your problems about making this desire, as your concerns is probably terrible to your intermittent fasting journey. So, what are the worries you have got approximately addressing this adventure? What wondering ought to make you prevent intermittent fasting? Here are a few troubles that want to be addressed.

• Breakfast is the maximum vital meal of the day, I can't miss it or bypass it — Well, newsflash! Breakfast is not the most essential meal of the day as dinner isn't always the maximum crucial meal of the night time time, every of them are certainly unbiased food and there's not something all too particular about it. So, sure, it's miles adequate to skip breakfast due to the fact in fact consuming breakfast obtained't fire up or increase the metabolism sports activities in your frame, and skipping breakfast received't make you advantage any greater weight.

• It's ok to go with snacks — It's in truth now not k to go with snacks. Snacking doesn't improve your metabolism and as such can not help you shed pounds. In fact, in step with the have a take a look at, snacking carefully contributes to fatty liver sickness and weight troubles.

• Fasting will sluggish down my metabolism – Well, that's absolutely the possibility of what fasting does for you. Intermittent fasting, in fact, permits you maintain extra muscle and will increase the extent of your metabolism even as, on the same time, allows you shed kilos. It's a win-win state of affairs.

So, deal with the ones issues and get prepared to begin intermittent fasting due to the fact if something at all, it's miles a big bonus in your fitness. Are you organized? Let's begin. As a Chinese proverb as fast as stated, "The temptation to quit can be finest just in advance than you're approximately to be triumphant." With that stated, press on and press on.

Day 1 – Don't eat after dinner

Whatever the temptation is, do now not eat after dinner. I may need to replicate that boldly, "DO NOT EAT AFTER DINNER!"

There, that's an awful lot higher! Eat a few element you normally devour at some point of the day however as speedy as it's after dinner, stop consuming. You ate dinner at 7 PM and don't experience definitely hungry round eight to 9 PM, however the second you watch TV, living room on the couch, or spend remarkable time with your family to lighten up and unwind, you begin feeling so hungry that you can eat the entire residence.

At this time, the alternatives to go for are within the most important snacks, ice cream, chips, or a few popcorn. They appearance pretty harmless and a outstanding preference, but they may be now not going to help you out of it. Here are suggestions to help you through the ordeal and through the night time time;

• Instead of eating meals or a snack, pick out having a heat cup of calming tea or natural tea or a tumbler of water.

• Brush out your teeth. As you sweep out your teeth, the minty taste will help to scale back all starvation pangs and cravings and additionally help you ship a subconscious message on your mind and your frame which you are completed consuming for the day. And if it doesn't agree with you, then you may have to brush it out once more. Trust me, it in reality works without a doubt well.

• Say goodnight and bypass proper to bed. Call it a night time time, you've eaten dinner and now it's time to hit the sack.

Day 2 – Stall Breakfast

It's a cute morning and bet what? You've definitely finished a 12-hour speedy. Isn't that brilliant? The very last meal you had grow to be dinner at 7 PM ultimate night time time and proper now, it's already 7 AM. That way you completed 12 hours of rapid and if my calculations are accurate, that means that you didn't devour for half of of of an afternoon. You've balanced your fasting and eating ratio to 50:50, 12 hours of fasting, and 12 hours of ingesting. That's a huge win and all you needed to do changed into halt ingesting sports after dinner and sleep via it.

But wait! It's the morning rush and it's hitting tough. You've have been given to leave the house on your place of work otherwise you're going to be past due, so what do you do? You devour something as fast as you may or take preserve of out some thing at the fly that you could munch in the vehicle. But why do all that? Why now not honestly stall breakfast nowadays, take maintain of a cup of tea, a cup of coffee, or a tumbler of water and wait to consume on the identical time because it's handy to?

As said in advance, there's now not something incorrect with stalling the primary meal of the day until it's available and until you've made the proper choice. It is crucial to pay attention to what precisely we placed into our stomachs in the course of breakfast. A handy time is probably moments whilst you've dropped the youngsters off at faculty and are once more domestic or when you've arrived at your place of business, each of those instances is handy to devour breakfast in vicinity of seeking out to get one amidst the morning rush.

Settle in whilst you've gotten to art work, test the calendar, and plan your day, after that, test your email and respond to them. Remember that during this time, you don't should have breakfast whilst you're wearing out the ones sports activities or sneak in breakfast. Just examine the ones steps:

• Wait till 10 AM. Now, that's it 10 AM, it's time to revel in some element you normally have for breakfast and this will be more thrilling as there may be no chaos.

• Don't rush for lunch at 12 noon. It's lunchtime already but you certainly had breakfast 2 hours inside the past, so there's each tendency which you're not truely that hungry. So, while the clock is announcing that it's time for lunch, your frame honestly tells you that it isn't. Wait till you sense pretty hungry before going for lunch.

• It's 2 PM already? Okay, it's time to have a pleasing lunch since you're probably feeling hungry. Enjoy your lunch.

• Finally, consume dinner at 7 PM.

Note: You already have a time table for intermittent fasting, so boom on the preceding steps. Don't devour after dinner and stall breakfast till 10 AM.

Day three – Say no to snacks!

Wow! You're three days in and also you've already long lengthy long gone on a 15-hour rapid. Last night time time, you had dinner at 7 PM, you didn't eat some factor after that, and then, you stalled breakfast till 10 AM. Here's the subsequent step, don't consume some element after lunch until dinner.

It's time to keep away from snacking and in reality sticking to consuming proper. Here are pointers to help you prevent or at excellent, keep away from snacking:

•   Remembering that dinner is just a few hours away and that you are in fact going to consume quick will assist you live a ways from snacking for a piece. All you want to do is expect a few moments earlier than succumbing to snacking.

•   Hunger craving and hunger pangs come in waves, if you permit it wash away after the primary wave without drowning in it, it loses its stress and subsides grade by grade. It's brief, it received't ultimate the whole day, so clearly permit it die out.

• Sometimes, hunger pangs and cravings aren't actual as you may no longer simply be hungry. It is viable that every one you experience is an aftermath of your afternoon snacking addiction or which you're genuinely simply thirsty. It can also be due to your emotions, if you're feeling bored, sad, worried, worrying, or burdened out, then you could have a compulsion to devour. Instead of accomplishing out for a snack to munch on, why no longer without a doubt have a pitcher of water, get a cup of espresso or tea, and down it. Trust me, it allows.

• Get your head back into your artwork. When you submerge your self into work, you forget about about each different human necessity besides respiratory. By the time you choose up the responsibilities, do more paintings, take a stroll, name a chum or a purchaser, perform a circle of relatives chore, you'll discover the starvation cravings and hunger pangs slowly dissipating and demise out. Before you understand it, you're meeting remaining dates, chatting for hours, taking element within the lovely environment, or finished with the chore and boom, it's time to transport home and enjoy dinner.

- Finally, consume dinner at 7 PM.

Note: You have already got a time desk for intermittent fasting, so building up on the previous steps. Don't devour after dinner and stall breakfast till 10 AM, and don't have any snacks between lunch and dinner.

Day four – Let's pass breakfast

That's it, as every day passes via, you've got got come to be one step within the path of the stop line. Just test your achievements, you completed a fifteen-hour fast and also you didn't for as speedy as succumb to snacking. Last night, you had dinner at 7 PM, you didn't consume something after that, after which, you stalled breakfast until 10 AM and didn't consume a few aspect between lunch and dinner. Here's the subsequent step, skip breakfast through ready one more hour. Yes, wait until 11 AM to eat and make lunch the primary meal of your day.

It's time to begin remembering each of those steps and repeating all the capabilities that you've been getting to know:

•   Mindful eating. This is the artwork of no longer consuming even as you're wearing out an interest.

• Not consuming due to the emotions that you're feeling, out of addiction, or at the same time as you're thirsty. You recognize higher now and that's why you handiest consume at the equal time as you certainly and in reality experience hungry.

• Remember that starvation is temporal, it's pretty brief-lived. This approach that it doesn't final for prolonged and as such want to no longer be rated as a task. Carry out the guidelines that will help you surf over the waves till they subside and fade away.

• Finally, consume dinner at 7 PM.

Note: You already have a time table for intermittent fasting, so increase at the previous steps. Don't devour after dinner and stall breakfast till eleven AM, and don't have any snacks amongst lunch and dinner. Every step counts and each step subjects, so use them properly.

Day 5 – Repeat

What's that I pay attention? You truely finished a 16-hour speedy? That's exceptional! You deserve an award. Congratulations! So, you had dinner very last night time at 7 PM, you stalled breakfast till 11 AM to devour your first meal, you didn't snack up and you didn't eat whatever till it became dinnertime at 7 PM.

Guess what? You've truely broken into an intermittent fasting protocol referred to as the sixteen/8 Intermittent Fasting Method. It changed into popularized with the useful resource of manner of Martin Berkhan and has severa versions. It's considered a well-known intermittent fasting method because it uses one key reality, the truth that it is simple to bypass breakfast due to the fact most parents aren't surely hungry inside the morning.

This moreover reduces your consuming time table or window to 1-zero.33 of the day this is eight hours. By doing this, you have got unfolded the window of possibilities to rapid to a whooping -1/3 of the day that is 16 hours. From right here on, the healing effects of intermittent fasting begin to kick in.

Now, it's time to start and repeat the techniques. Stall breakfast and go away snacking out maximum of the window frame of lunch and dinner and don't eat after dinner. Stick to the plan you first had in the starting, don't consume after dinner and stall breakfast till eleven AM, and don't take any snacks among lunch and dinner. Every step counts and each step topics, so use them properly.

Fasting is a high-quality tool for enhancing your health and dropping weight, maximum of the time, it's far an lousy lot better than simply eating a low carbohydrate and excessive-fats weight loss program. But it's miles essential to word that it obtained't paintings, similar to all others gained't if you don't do it constantly and successfully. It all relies upon on how nicely you do it. So, in case you see yourself slipping up, embody it, start once more from day one, or try to pick up from in that you slipped, it will immensely do you a whole lot of suitable.

Still now not quality if intermittent fasting is for you? Here are some experts that will help you decide:

• It's a good deal simpler and easier to stick to intermittent fasting due to the truth, on a everyday day, you pass food each time you're too busy to eat or no longer hungry.

• It can without difficulty be geared up into your life-style. You don't must go through drastic changes to start intermittent fasting.

• It will help combat the cravings and pangs of starvation whether or not actual or fake. Intermittent fasting helps you to boom the talents had to enjoy out the flow and waves of hunger via the usage of making you switch out to be extra aware about the reasons you devour.

Sometimes, you don't must see the entire staircase before you are taking step one and when you start stepping, maintain on going, difficult, and strong.

Chapter 20: How To Use Intermittent Fasting Successfully

Since the start of this ebook, you've been reading so many things about how intermittent fasting is a wonderful intervention for losing weight and living a healthful lifestyles. Let's simply say that you picked up this ebook so that you can shed the greater pounds that you have picked up inside the path of the lockdown duration.

Whatever made you select out up the ebook doesn't without a doubt depend quantity proper now as hundreds as you ensuring which you do it effectively. Intermittent fasting first grabbed the eye of developing old and metabolism researchers and clinicians even as it have end up an opportunity to non-prevent caloric limit, earlier than in the end turning into no longer only an extremely good weight loss possibility however additionally a lift to as a minimum one's metabolic fitness.

At the prevent of 2020 and into 2021, you is probably looking for to have a wonderful "beach frame," stave off growing older and metabolic sickness, or probably, you truly need to sense alive and healthful, strolling round collectively together with your youngsters and grandchildren. Intermittent fasting will let you attain every and each one of these goals but it's far critical to recollect that one time desk of intermittent fasting doesn't healthy all of us. You want to keep in thoughts your goals and strength wishes into attention to apply intermittent fasting correctly. You will need to go to your dietician, scientific nutritionist, and the physician to make sure that it sincerely works out nicely.

Getting Started with Intermittent Fasting

Intermittent fasting is an umbrella term to classify pretty some eating strategies and schedules to on and rancid calorie rules. It includes a weekly or each day cycle of feeding and fasting. The famous and maximum commonplace intermittent fasting strategies consist of the following; the five:2 food regimen which includes 2 fasting days in which you eat nothing greater than 500 power in keeping with day, the trade-day fasting which incorporates eating fewer than 500 energy on selected days, and the time-constrained feeding, which the well-known one is the sixteen:eight hours ration of fasting to feeding. The sixteen:eight time-restricted feeding consists of you consuming inside a time-body of eight hours and fasting for eight hours. Other time-constrained feedings may additionally additionally contain you having a feeding window for 6 to 12 hours each day and fasting for 12 hours to 18 hours or more every day.

If you're beginning out with intermittent fasting, it's far drastically endorsed to start slowly. Slowly artwork as a whole lot because the fasting schedule goal over the path of weeks, months, or years. Start out first with a prolonged overnight fasting length of 12 hours or greater every day and from there, begin to work up your manner to fourteen or sixteen hours so that you can trouble in a mean each day time-restricted feeding pattern. From there, you could flow into directly to fasting for extended hours of 24 to forty eight hours on a weekly or monthly basis. You really want to bear in mind this, choose a time table that suits together with your health goals.

How to apply Intermittent Fasting for Weight Loss

How masses weight you lose in some unspecified time in the future of your intermittent fasting completely relies upon on you and the method which you use. Studies display that it takes at least no a great deal less than to three months and a maximum of six months to lose 10 pounds using the alternate-day fasting or five:2 weight loss plan.

Factor in while you consume, what your each day requirements are, and the way you begin will determine exactly how a top notch deal you'll lose. Intermittent fasting schedules will help limit your calorie intake definitely and sell you dropping weight hastily. Combining it with extra calorie restrict and more healthy food options with intermittent fasting will assist accelerate your weight loss program.

Tips for Losing Weight with Intermittent Fasting

• Increase your fiber intake. Increasing your fiber intake amongst food will enhance the fitness of your gut and satiety.

• Stick in your fasting calorie dreams.

• Avoid ingesting too many power-dense snacks and food for your change everyday non-fast days.

•   Increase your intake of lean protein. This will help decorate your muscle businesses and satiety and help you shed kilos with reduced hunger over a prolonged term.

•   Eat plenty in advance rather than later. Eating at some point of the night or past due at night time prevents your body from burning fats due to the truth it's far near bedtime. Everyone has an inner clock which allows regulate our body. It's an inexperienced tool that switches from usually the usage of carbohydrates subsequently of the day for energy to via and massive using fats in the course of the night time, but it is able to detrimentally go off whilst you unbalance it with a middle of the night snack. By eating past due, your frame kicks into burning carbohydrates while it is meant to be burning fat.

www.ingramcontent.com/pod-product-compliance
Lightning Source LLC
Chambersburg PA
CBHW071338120626
46546CB00002B/605